Do Go Gentle

ALSO BY CHRISTOPHER STOOKEY

FICTION
Terminal Care
Where Death Is a Hunter

Do Go Gentle

Bringing My Father Home to Die With Dignity After a Devastating Stroke

Christopher Stookey

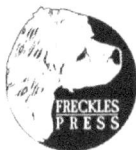

FRECKLES
PRESS

DO GO GENTLE

Copyright © 2015 by Christopher Stookey

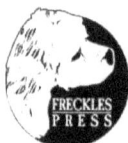

First printing May 2015
10 9 8 7 6 5 4 3 2 1

ISBN-13: 978-0692433751
ISBN-10:   0692433759

Book Design by Andrea Orlic

In memory of my father and mother

And to George, with thanks

Author's note: This is a true story. However, with the exception of members of my immediate family and close friends, names have been changed to protect the privacy of the individuals involved.

PREFACE

On a fall night while in his bed at home, my father suffered a massive stroke that left him paralyzed and unable to communicate. After several days in the hospital intensive care unit, and after a series of scans and other tests, his doctors pronounced a grim prognosis: recovery was highly unlikely. My immediate family—my mother, my sister, and I—were faced with a very difficult decision: should we place Dad in a nursing home and, using a feeding tube, keep him alive as long as possible? Or should we forego the feeding tube and bring him home—to die?

This is the story of our decision to bring Dad home.

I wrote this book because I wanted to describe my family's experience with the planned death of a loved one at home on hospice. California, the state where my father died, does not allow "assisted dying." At the time of this writing, five states—Oregon, Washington, Vermont, Montana, and New Mexico—allow terminally ill individuals the choice to hasten death by means of doctor-assisted dying. Because assisted death was not available in California, my father died a "natural death" owing to dehydration, that is, a death brought about by the withholding of all food and water. Dying for him took place over several days in his bed at home. This book describes that dying process in a frank and honest manner.

I also wrote this book because I wanted to increase awareness about stroke, the third most common cause of death in the United States. About 800,000 people suffer a stroke each year in the US; 15 million worldwide. A person living in the United States today has a one in six chance of someday having a stroke. My father was a victim of those odds.

Finally, I wrote this book for my father. In telling the story of his death, I also tell the story of his life. I hope that readers of this book will come to know him a little, and something of his life will be preserved on these pages. For me, he was bigger than life; he was the man who brought me into the world and the father who loved me beyond measure. This book is, then, is a final goodbye to him, a final act of love.

CS

Table of Contents

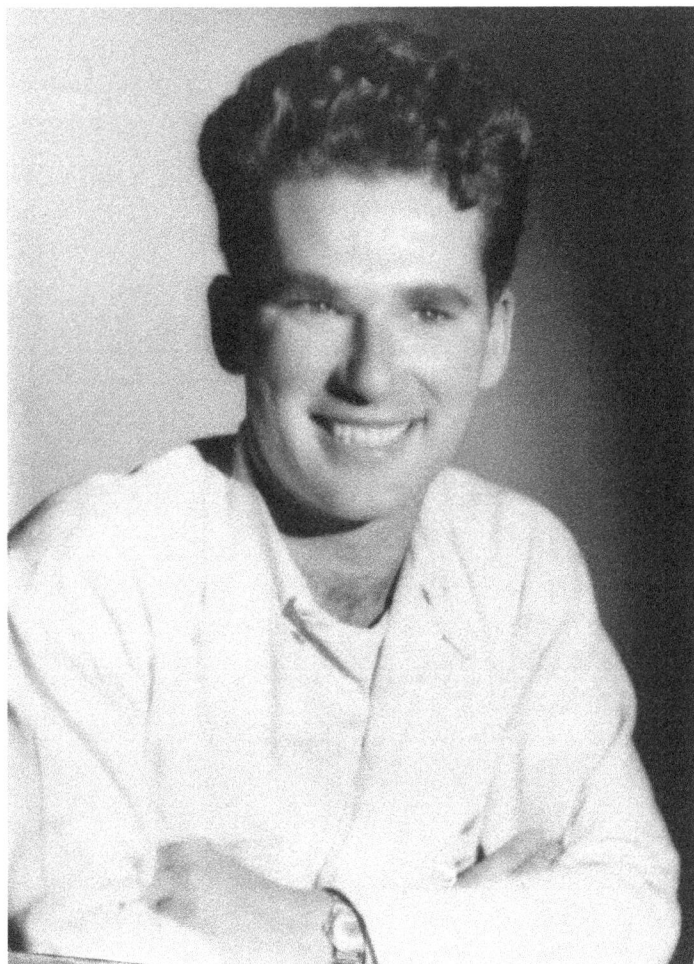

Do Go Gentle

I. Thunderbolt

On a warm, sunny Southern California morning in early September, my mother walked into her bedroom and found her husband, my eighty-three-year-old father, lying face up on the floor next to the bed. He was making odd movements with his left arm and ineffectual, pedaling motions with his left leg. My mother's initial reaction was one of annoyance. "Bill," she said, "what in the world are you doing there on the floor?"

However, her irritation quickly turned into concern. My father appeared to be trying to get up, but he couldn't. Moreover, he was trying to say something, but his speech was severely garbled, the words unintelligible. My mom tried to help my father to his feet, but it was no use. She began to panic.

She rushed to the phone and tried to call me, her physician son, at home. She should have known I'd be at work, but she wasn't thinking terribly clearly. My wife, Sandy, answered the phone, and my mom explained the situation. Sandy made the obvious response: call 911. She assured my mother she would call me at work, but the first thing to do was to get my father to the hospital. Immediately.

Sandy phoned me at work and explained the situation. I called Mom as soon as I could pull away from the patient I was seeing. When I reached her, she said the paramedics had already arrived. "They think your father's having a stroke," she said.

"Oh God! Sounds like it, yes," I said.

Mom told me they were taking my dad to St. Mark's, the nearest hospital to my parents' house, located about three miles away. "When they put him on the stretcher," she said, "he kept saying, 'No, no.' It's hard to understand him, but I don't think he wants to go to the hospital."

"Well, he has no choice," I said. "I'll meet you at St. Mark's. I'll leave work. Someone will cover for me."

"They said it might be a stroke," my mom repeated, forgetting she'd just told me this.

"See you at the hospital," I said.

The drive to St. Mark's took me about an hour. When I arrived at the emergency room, I checked in as a family member. I was wearing hospital scrubs, and it must have looked strange, my standing there in line wearing hospital attire. Several people gave me puzzled looks.

They took me back to the stretcher area and told me my dad was in the last bed on the right. The first thing I saw was Mom sitting in a chair against a wall located several yards from Dad's bed. She looked so alone and out of place sitting there—apparently she didn't understand that she could move her chair next to my father's bed. I grabbed her hands. She stood up, and we hugged.

"They think he's having a stroke," my mom said once again.

"Let me take a look," I said. "Come on with me."

"No, I'll sit down. You go."

I went to Dad's bedside. He was lying on his back propped up on one side by pillows, oxygen tubing in his nose, an IV dripping in his forearm. Immediately, a sinking feeling came over me. His face was drooping noticeably on the right side, and the right corner of his mouth was pulled down in a contorted half-frown. His eyes were fixed in an unnatural gaze upward and to the left. His right arm and leg lay unnaturally atop additional pillows, and it was obvious he couldn't move the right side of his body. My legs went rubbery. It was a

16

stroke, all right, and it was a bad one. I positioned myself at the side of the bed in the direction his eyes were pointing, so he could see me—assuming he could see at all. In doing so, I noted a flicker of expression on the left, non-droopy, side of his face. It seemed he recognized me. He was able to move his eyes a little; he could bring them almost to look straight forward, but he could not look to the right.

"Hey," I said squeezing his right hand. "Hey." It was the only thing I could think of to say.

He made an attempt to speak, a movement of the mouth followed by an unintelligible sound. However, he could not talk. My father, never in his life at a loss for words, could not talk.

Then he coughed, and a small trickle of saliva ran out the right corner of his mouth. You could see he was having trouble swallowing as well. My stomach twisted. I grabbed a paper towel from a dispenser on the wall and wiped the saliva from his mouth.

Tossing the paper towel in the trash, I slipped my fingers into the palm of my dad's right hand. "Can you squeeze?" I asked. "Squeeze my hand!" Again, there was a hint of expression, a flicker of comprehension, on the left side of his face. However, he did not squeeze. The hand was completely lifeless and limp. I lifted his entire right arm off the bed—it was flaccid. I gently set the arm back down on the pillow. "Can you wiggle your toes?" I asked squeezing his right foot under the blanket. "Wiggle." Again, no movement. The entire right side of his body, from his face to his toes, was paralyzed.

Next, I slipped my fingers into his left hand and, again, asked him to squeeze. He *was* able to make a weak squeeze with the left hand. "There you go, good," I said lifting up his left arm. Unlike the flaccid right arm, there was some muscle tone, but it was still very weak. The same was true of the left leg. He could move his leg slightly, but not enough to lift it off the bed.

I was puzzled. Usually a stroke affects just one side of the body. Dad was obviously completely paralyzed on the right, but he was also very weak on the left. Bilateral involvement. Unable to speak. Unable to swallow. I'd been working as an emergency physician for nearly twenty years, and I'd seen a lot of patients with strokes. This was one of the worst I'd ever seen.

I adjusted the pillow under his head as well as the pillows supporting his right arm. "I'm going over to talk to Mom," I said. "She's right here, sitting in a chair. I'll be right back. We're both here."

I went over and sat down next to my mom. She'd been watching me with Dad, but she had not come to the bedside with me. Honestly, at that moment, she didn't look strong enough to stand on her own. She appeared to be in a state of shock.

"Definitely a stroke," I said. "It seems to be mainly on the right side. There's still some strength on the left." I was trying to say something positive. "He squeezed my hand."

"He did?" Mom said. "Is that good?"

Just then, the ER doctor walked up. He was a young Asian man, probably in his mid-thirties, wearing surgical scrubs and a white coat. I stood up and introduced myself. Although I had not identified myself as a physician, he addressed me as "doctor." I suppose my own surgical scrubs were a clue, and my mom probably told him her "doctor son" was on the way. "The CT scan shows no signs of bleeding," the doctor said. "That's good, but unfortunately, we don't know when the stroke began. Your mother found him on the floor this morning, so it could have occurred anytime during the night. He can't talk and tell us when the weakness started. So we can't give TPA because we don't know if we're inside or outside the three-hour window."

The "three-hour window" the doctor was referring to was the time limit for giving "TPA," a clot-busting drug. There are two types of strokes: one caused by bleeding in the brain, the other caused by a blood clot in the brain. My dad's CT scan had shown no signs of brain bleeding; therefore, he must have had the blood clot type of stroke. However, TPA must be given within three hours after the stroke starts; otherwise, it's of no use. If it's given after three hours, it's not only ineffective, it can have lethal side effects. Since we didn't know when the stroke had started, the doctor couldn't give the TPA. It would be too dangerous. In other words, Dad had had a stroke, a very bad stroke—and there was nothing anyone could do about it.

The doctor told me an ultrasound study of my dad's heart (checking for blood clots—stroke-causing clots often originate in the heart) had been ordered. After the ultrasound, Dad would be moved to the ICU. The doctor said we were free to stay with him as long as we wished, but the ultrasound test and the transfer to the ICU would take a couple hours. Perhaps, the doctor suggested, my mother and I might want to take a break and have some lunch while they did the ultrasound. The ICU nurse would call us when my father had settled into the ICU.

I gave the doctor my cell phone number and thanked him. I liked him. He'd been polite and professional. He'd told me everything I needed to know—even though the news he'd delivered was bad news. After the doctor left, Mom and I went back to Dad's bedside. I pulled Mom's chair over so she could

19

sit down next to the bed. She hadn't understood a word the doctor had said, but that was okay. She wasn't asking many questions right now anyway. I positioned her chair so she was in my father's leftward field of vision. "Hold his left hand," I said. "He can feel you on that side. He can see you and hear you. He understands."

I pulled up another chair for myself. "They're going to do an ultrasound test," I said to my dad. "Looking for blood clots." He looked back at me, and there was a slight movement of his lips. I decided against any further explanation of the ultrasound test; even if they found clots in his heart, there wasn't much they could do about it, anyway (they weren't going to open up his heart and remove the clots).

My mom held my dad's hand and stroked his half-paralyzed face. She didn't say much. It's hard to know what to say to someone who can't talk back to you. So, for the next half hour, we simply sat with him. From time to time, I wiped away the saliva that dripped from the corner of his mouth. His eyes remained open, and occasionally he would cough.

I wondered how much *he* understood about what was happening. Did he even know he'd had a stroke? Should I tell him? Should I try to explain? I decided to say nothing. It seemed the best plan for now. Besides, I didn't feel like wearing my doctor's hat at that moment. Like Mom, I was feeling a bit overwhelmed—I would leave the explaining to his doctors.

To tell the truth, I think at that moment I was somewhat in a state of shock, myself. This was my father lying there before me, the man who had always been the pillar of strength in my life. Now he was helpless as an infant. The idea of his being conscious yet barely able to move or speak or even to swallow—it was almost too hard to think about. Irrationally,

20

my gut impulse was to rip the IV out in his arm, remove the oxygen tubing from his nose, and walk him out of the ER and take him home. Everything would be okay when we got him home. Somehow, everything would be okay if we could just get him back home.

Of course, everything would not be okay, and I did not rip out Dad's IV. Instead, I sat there with Mom at the bedside, and we took turns holding his hand. We spoke to him a little: "Do you want me to adjust the pillow? Are the lights too bright?" It was all we could do just then. Be with him, touch him, comfort him, let him know he was not alone.

*   *   *

When they took him away for the ultrasound, Mom and I went for lunch at a restaurant a couple of blocks away. We could have gone to the hospital cafeteria, but we both wanted to get out of the hospital for a little while.

I don't think Mom took more than two bites of her food; her hand trembled as she drank her glass of water. Both her parents had died from complications of stroke. She understood the seriousness of her husband's condition.

She explained to me, once again, how she'd found Dad on the bedroom floor in the morning. She'd fallen asleep on the couch watching a movie and had slept, as she sometimes does, all night long on the couch. Dad had gone to bed at around 10:00. He'd seemed perfectly fine. She had no idea how long he'd been on the floor.

She commented again about how he had seemed to say "No" over and over as the paramedics took him away. "He never liked hospitals," she said. "I think he's afraid he might go in and never come out alive." Then she fell silent. Her eyes

21

welled up with tears. I knew what she was thinking: *Maybe he wouldn't.*

I finished most of my meal while my mom sat and stared blankly at her plate. I realized my sister, Lori, who also lives nearby in Southern California, had not yet been informed of what had happened. I phoned her, but she was at work and did not answer. I left a message with her message service. "Dad's in the emergency room at St. Mark's. He's had a stroke. I'm afraid it's pretty bad."

*   *   *

When we got back to the ER, my father was no longer there. He'd been transferred to the ICU on the fourth floor. No one had yet called me on my cell phone; we got the information from the ER clerk. We rode the elevator upstairs and entered the ICU waiting room. An elderly woman, a volunteer wearing a pink uniform, sat at a desk in front of a locked door. Her job was to call back to the nurses when visitors arrived and to ask if it was okay for visitors to come in. We identified ourselves and the volunteer called back. She said it was okay for us to go in; he was in Bed 5.

We entered the ICU unescorted. Mom looked frightened as we walked down the hall, moving through the unfamiliar surroundings. I asked a nurse which way to Room 5, and she gave us directions. I was still wearing my scrubs, and it felt strange to be in the ICU as a visitor. We passed by the nursing station. The nurses and doctors were there going about their business. It was just another day at the hospital for them; no one paid attention to us. We walked past the patient rooms, small suites with sliding glass doors. In nearly all the rooms, the curtains were fully open, and the patients inside were in full view. Some looked very sick; several were on ventilator life support. Other patients, however, hardly seemed ill at all; they were sitting up in bed watching TV or chatting with visitors.

Near the end of the hall, we came to Room 5. I put my arm around Mom. "Here we are," I said. We stepped in front of the glass, and there was my father, lying in the bed in the middle of the otherwise unoccupied room. He was facing the window, propped up on his right side the same way he'd been propped up in the ER. Although he was facing toward us, I could see his eyes were still held in that left-upward gaze. He appeared to be looking up at the ceiling.

We entered the room. I walked to the side of the bed and took his left hand. "Hey. They moved you upstairs. How are you doing?"

As before, Dad tried to speak, but he was only able to make weak, unintelligible sounds.

Mom and I switched places. "Hi, Bill," she said. "Are you feeling any better?"

While she stroked Dad's hand and talked to him, I looked at the monitor screens above his bed. His vital signs were all normal: blood pressure and pulse, heart rhythm, oxygen level. The oxygen tubing was still anchored in his nose, and the IV was still dripping into his forearm. I looked up at the TV on the wall above the bed—it was playing an afternoon talk show, but the sound was turned off.

Just as I started to wonder where Dad's nurse was, a young woman in teal scrubs walked into the room. She had a stethoscope draped around her neck, and her dark brown hair was pinned up in a bun. She entered the room without saying hello or introducing herself. She strode to the computer mounted on a stand next to the bed and began typing. After a minute of watching her type, I began to feel annoyed at how

23

she was completely ignoring us. I cleared my throat and said, "Hi. I'm Chris, Mr. Stookey's son. Are you his nurse?" Of course, I knew she *was* Dad's nurse.

The nurse looked up as if noticing us for the first time. "Yes," she said. "You are…?"

"Chris, his son, and Betty Stookey, his wife." I was put off by the nurse's curtness. No introductions, no hello. "How's he doing?" I asked a bit pointedly.

"Have you talked to the doctor?" the nurse asked.

"No," I said. "We just got here. We did talk to the ER doctor downstairs."

"Dr. Preston was here. Dr. Sims is the neurologist."

"Dr. Preston—he's…?"

"The admitting doctor."

"Will he be coming by again?"

"He was here half an hour ago."

I took this to mean Dr. Preston would not be coming by again—at least not anytime soon. "And Dr. Sims?"

"He's the neurologist."

"Yes, that's what you said. Will he be coming?"

"He saw your father down in the ER."

The nurse then picked up a bar code reader—a gun-like devise—and used it to read the bar code on the IV bag hanging above my father's bed. She returned to her typing. Bedside manner was not her forte.

Then, suddenly—as though a switch had been flipped on—the nurse turned to us and launched into a long series of questions about my father's past medical history. "Does Mr. Stookey have any health problems?" she asked. She directed her questions to Mom who, in turn, looked at me for help.

"Heart attack fifteen years ago," I said. "He had coronary artery bypass surgery shortly after that."

The nurse typed. "Heart attack fifteen years ago, bypass surgery. Okay. Respiratory? Lung problems?"

"No," I said.

"Smoker?"

"Quit when he had the heart attack."

"Alcohol?"

"A couple drinks a day. Sometimes a bit more."

"Allergies?"

"Penicillin," I said. I kept my answers short, in line with the tone of the questions. Dad's medical history wasn't terribly complicated. He'd been in good health until about age sixty-seven when he'd had a small heart attack. At the time, he was a heavy smoker, two or three packs a day. He quit smoking and underwent a quadruple coronary artery bypass operation. The operation had gone well, and he'd had no further heart trouble. A decade later, he was diagnosed with prostate cancer. He underwent radiation treatment, and, again, the results were good. His only other medical problem—until now—was arthritis of the knees.

"Is he taking medication?" the nurse asked.

"Aspirin," I said. "One baby aspirin a day as a blood thinner."

"Anything else?"

"Tylenol sometimes," Mom added. "For his knees."

The nurse typed on her computer. "Is that it?"

"Yes," I said.

The nurse moved on to a new set of questions, once again directing the questions to my mom, even though I was providing most of the answers.

"Does Mr. Stookey have an advance directive?"

Mom turned to me with a blank look.

"It's a legal document," I said, explaining to Mom. "It

tells the doctors what you—what he—wants done if he can't make decisions for himself anymore." I looked at the nurse. "I'm almost sure he has one."

"Did you bring it with you?" the nurse asked.

Obviously we hadn't. I looked at Mom. "Do you know where he keeps it?"

"No, I never—"

"That's going to be important," the nurse interrupted. "Given his condition."

"There's a binder with his important papers at home," I said. "I'll look for it."

"Do *you* know what his wishes are?" the nurse asked. "In case something happens. For example, if he stops breathing, would he want to be placed on a respirator?"

Mom turned to me, looking very perplexed.

"We'll look for the directive," I said.

"What do *you* want done?" the nurse asked my mother.

I knew it was a question Mom couldn't answer. I didn't know the answer either, at least not with certainty. Dad and I had never talked about his wishes in the case of a medical emergency. I had my suspicions, however, regarding what he would want—or, rather, what he would not want. My dad was not a keep-me-alive-at-all-costs kind of person. He had a philosophical, resigned attitude toward death. "I don't think he would want his life prolonged artificially," I said to the nurse.

"So…that's a 'no' on the respirator?"

"I don't…we'll have to look for the directive." I looked at Dad. We were having this conversation in front of him as though he were not even present in the room. He lay there expressionlessly, staring up at the ceiling. I wondered how much he heard and understood.

"What if his heart stops beating?" the nurse asked.

26

"Would he want his heart shocked, chest compressions?"

Mom looked at me with a combination of alarm and bewilderment.

"We'll find the directive," I said. "In the meantime, let's just say do everything possible till we know more."

The nurse frowned. Apparently, this was not the answer she was looking for. She typed on her computer, then moved on to her next set of questions. "Does he have a primary doctor?" she asked.

"Yes, Dr. Wilber," Mom said.

"Wilber?" the nurse said. She typed on her keyboard. "Is that one 'l' or two?"

*   *   *

After the nurse finished her questions, she left. Alone in the room, we sat with Dad into the afternoon. At one point, a pair of orderlies came in, and they "turned" him, repositioning him from his right side onto his left side. The repositioning, I knew, was done in order to prevent bedsores. Since Dad couldn't move the right side of his body, he needed to be shifted every couple hours, propped one side up with pillows.

As they were leaving, I asked the orderlies if they thought the neurologist would be in to talk to us. They said they didn't know, but that the doctors usually rounded on patients in the morning. At least this was something—it was more information than I'd gotten from the ICU nurse.

Toward the late afternoon, Dad drifted off to sleep. I don't know if he'd been given any sort of sedative or not. At 6:00 PM, the ICU nurse came in and told us they closed down visiting hours from 6:00 to 7:00 in order to clean the rooms and the halls. We were welcome to come back at 7:00.

Mom and I decided to go home, with the plan to return early the next morning and catch the doctors on their rounds. We left without waking Dad, who seemed to be sleeping pretty peacefully—better to let him sleep, we agreed. Mom kissed him gently on the cheek and said, "Be back soon, Honey. Tomorrow morning. See you then. I love you."

I lightly stroked his forehead with the back of my hand and whispered, "Get some rest, Dad. See ya tomorrow."

We started out, but Mom had left her purse under her chair. I went back, grabbed it, and walked back to the door where she stood. I put my arm around her shoulder, and we headed home.

II. The Life

William (Bill) Chapman Stookey was born on August 8th, 1925, in the small town of Marshall, Michigan (located on "the thumb" of Michigan). An only child, his parents were poor. His father, George Stookey, made a living working various odd jobs ranging from handyman to vacuum cleaner salesman. When the Depression hit in 1929, George struggled greatly to support the family. Billy remembered times when he went to bed hungry.

He had a difficult time in school. He had a learning disability (I suspect the problem was dyslexia, but a formal diagnosis was never made), and he was put in the remedial class, or "the retarded class," as my dad called it. However, when he reached the forth or fifth grade, one of his teachers, a Mrs. Mumby, concluded he didn't really belong in the remedial class, and she worked with him to bring him back into the regular class. Dad would always remember this, and later in life he established the "Vida Mumby Appreciation Fund," a charitable fund that donated money to the Marshall, Michigan school system.

As the Depression deepened, Dad's family moved west, looking for work. They landed in Washington State, in the town of Tacoma where George Stookey found employment as an office clerk. Dad liked Tacoma. He especially loved to hunt and fish (taking along his dog, a springer spaniel named "Ginger") in the woods surrounding their home. Sometimes the game he brought home would help put dinner on the table.

When Dad reached high school age, he started working in earnest to help support the family. He got a job as a message boy in the Tacoma shipyards. He worked the swing shift, going directly from school to the shipyards and putting in eight hours, five days a week. After his shift, he would often sleep on the ships, then return to school in the morning without ever having gone home. He said he had no trouble sleeping on the ships, despite the deafening hammering and riveting noises in the yard.

When he was a junior in high school, his mother became very ill. "Some sort of female cancer," he told me, unable to be more specific. His mother's gradual deterioration and her eventual death made a strong impact on Dad. He never talked about it much, but he would occasionally speak of the horror of her illness, referring to her swollen belly, the jaundice, the bedsores, and the gangrene that developed in her feet. For the rest of his life, Dad feared cancer. He once said to me in a moment of reflection, "All I know is I never want to die the way my mom died."

At seventeen, he lied about his age, saying he was a year older, and he signed up with the US Navy. It was 1942, and the United States had just become involved in World War II. Dad signed up with every intention of going to war as a sailor. As it turned out, however, the Navy had other plans for him. As part of the induction process, he had to take an IQ test, and to everyone's surprise (including my dad's), he scored high. The Navy decided to send him, not to war, but to college.

Dad, who'd never had any plans of going to college, humorously describes how he was given fifteen minutes to decide on a career path. After getting the results of the IQ test, an officer took him into a room and said, "The Navy is going to send you to college, Stookey. What do you want to study?"

"Well...I...I don't know. I never really thought about it."

"That's all right," the officer said, and he handed Dad a piece of paper. "Here's a list of the areas of study the Navy will support you through. Look it over. Take all the time you need. I'll be back in fifteen minutes for your decision."

Dad looked over the list: chemist, physicist, mechanical engineer, civil engineer…. Civil engineer. Building bridges, roads, canals, dams. That one sounded good. He'd always liked building things. The officer came back in the room, and my dad said he'd made his decision. He wanted to be a civil engineer. "Excellent," the officer said. "Good choice. Now, let's find you a college."

They ended up sending him to the California Institute of Technology in Southern California. Cal Tech. He had never heard of it. The induction officer told him it was a good school. The boy from the "retarded class" was headed for college in California.

During his second year at Cal Tech, family tragedy hit again. George Stookey, Dad's father, committed suicide by cutting his wrists. I don't know much about the details. If Dad was reluctant to talk about the death of his mother, he was even less willing to talk about his father's death. There were hints that, prior to his suicide, George had himself become ill. Dad once said during a dinner conversation, "After what my mother went through, I don't blame Dad for what he did." I didn't question the meaning of this at the time, but thinking about it now, I wonder if my grandfather also had a terminal illness—perhaps another case of cancer—and he didn't want to suffer the way his wife had suffered.

My dad was now an orphan—no mother, no father, no siblings—and the Navy became his surrogate family. He made it through his bachelor's degree and graduated in 1946. The war had just ended, and Dad missed shipping out to the Pacific theatre by a few months. Over the next four years, the newly-minted Ensign Stookey fulfilled his military obligation working as a Navy Seabee, designing and building storage depots to house the huge amount of equipment (tanks, Jeeps, trucks, airplanes, etc.) returning from the Pacific. He was stationed at Port Hueneme, California, south of Santa Barbara.

These were good years for Dad. The work was easy and not very closely supervised. He even learned to fly in his spare time and purchased a used, two-seater airplane, allegedly for $50. Living on the ocean, he also became an avid swimmer, and he became part of a Navy swim team that gave public performances (their big trick was swimming under large oil slicks that had been set on fire).

Dad liked to tell the story of how, in 1946, he became the first person to privately own and operate a four-wheel-drive vehicle. As the equipment piled up at Port Hueneme, there just wasn't enough space for it all. The inventory process for the equipment was horrible—no one had any idea how many Jeeps and trucks there were at the port. So, one day, in broad daylight, my dad just drove one of the vehicles home. No one cared. It was a four-cylinder, flat head, Willys Jeep. My dad claimed, in all seriousness, that he was the first private Jeep "owner" in America. He might have been right about that.

The most important event of those years, however, was undoubtedly the night he met his future wife, my mom, at a Navy dance in Los Angeles. Her name was Betty Dudney, and she was a pretty, brunette farm girl from Nebraska. Her family, like his, had come west looking for work, and she was working as a typist for the Southern California Gas Company. My parents say it was love at first sight.

I've seen pictures of my mom and dad during their dating days; they made a striking couple, my mom slim and attractive with her red painted lips, my dad handsome with his curly dark-brown hair and wearing his officer's uniform.

Dad made frequent trips down to LA from Port Hueneme for their dates. Sometimes he would drive down in his Jeep; sometimes he would fly. Once, and only once, he talked Mom into going up in his airplane. Of course, he had to show off, making banked turns and steep ascents. My mom swore she would never fly again.

The four-year military obligation neared an end, and Dad decided to continue his education and pursue a master's degree in civil engineering. The Navy was willing to foot the bill. He applied to MIT and was accepted to the graduate program there. He and Mom talked about how being apart would be difficult. Just before leaving for the East, Dad made one last flight in his plane. He flew over and "buzzed" the house where Mom lived with her parents in LA. She says he flew so low, she could see the white of his smile as he waved goodbye.

During the winter school winter break, my mom joined Dad in Boston. They toured New England, went down to New York City, and visited Washington, DC. On December 27th, 1950, they made it official. I don't know if they'd planned all along to get married or if they just decided on a lark. They tied the knot in the Roanoke, Virginia County Courthouse, in the office of the justice of the peace.

*   *   *

Dad finished his master's degree, and he and Mom moved back to Southern California. He settled into his first job as a civilian civil engineer, working for the Los Angeles Department of Water and Power. Although he was now free of his obligations to the Navy, he stayed on with the Seabees as a reservist. Once a month, he would put on his Navy uniform and spend the weekend working for the Navy as a construction engineer. Despite wars in Korea and Vietnam, he was never called to active duty. When he finally retired from the Navy twenty years later, he had reached the rank of Commander; he retired with full benefits.

I was born in 1955, the first child. Shortly thereafter, Dad took a new job as city engineer for the city of Fullerton in Orange County. My parents bought a home in Fullerton—a modest three-bedroom house located on the outskirts of town, surrounded by orange groves. This is the house they would live in for the rest of their lives.

Dad worked for Fullerton for seven years, building roads, bridges, underpasses, and flood systems. He worked long hours, often attending city council and planning commission meetings in the evening. He spent his non-Navy weekends doing work projects around the house. He built—by himself— a flagstone patio in the backyard with a brick fireplace, smoke oven, and brick barbeque. Other projects included brick planters in the front and backyards and a koi pond with a fountain in the backyard. He loved these projects, especially the brick work. When I look at his craftsmanship today (all of his projects are still standing), it's clear: he was a good mason.

I said my dad did these home projects by himself. That's not completely true. *I* helped him with the barbeque and the brick planters. I well remember driving in the open-air Jeep to the supply yard with him and watching the yard worker load sand with a tractor scoop into the trailer. I remember the smell of the fresh cement mixing in the mixer. Dad would assign me small tasks like wetting down the bricks or holding one end of a chalk line. When a project was finished, he would give me full credit despite the insignificance of my participation. The backyard planters were always, "The planters Chris and I made." The barbeque was, "The barbeque Chris and I built."

My sister, Lori, was born in 1962. It was the year of the Cuban Missile Crisis; John Glenn had become the first American to orbit the Earth; John Kennedy was president. I recall that Dad and I (I was now in second grade) took summer vacation alone that year and the next. We went backpacking in the Mineral King area of Sequoia National Park, hiking deep into the woods and sleeping under the stars. We caught trout at Eagle Lake and cooked the fish over a campfire. Leaning against our sleeping bags, we ate trout and canned beans and watched the shooting stars in the night sky. Dad, who always had a great interest in astronomy and science in general, told me the "shooting stars" weren't stars at all; they were rocks burning up in the atmosphere as they fell to Earth. Sometimes, he said, the rocks didn't completely burn up, and they fell all the way to the ground. I asked if the rocks ever hit people. "No, almost never. Usually the rocks just hit the ground or, more likely, they fall into the ocean."

I asked if the rocks made a big splash when they landed in the ocean.

"Oh yes," he said. "Sure, the big ones do. Sure."

*   *   *

Dad liked his work as city engineer, but over time he started to want more. He began dreaming of forming his own engineering company. Independence was in his blood, and it was perhaps inevitable he would want to head off on his own some day.

In 1964, he took the leap. He and a friend, a fellow civil engineer named Walter Thein, founded Willdan Associates, an independent civil engineering firm headquartered in Anaheim, California. "Headquarters" was a 12' X 30' trailer situated on a

35

vacant lot located about a mile away from Disneyland.

The early Willdan days were stressful for Dad. Even at age nine, I could see the signs of tension: the waking up at night, the pacing through the house, the chain-smoking of Marlboro cigarettes. I suspect he had sunk every dime we had into the business; he was risking everything. If he'd worked long hours at Fullerton, his hours were even longer now. He would usually leave for work when I was just getting up in the morning for school, and he would get back home just as I was going to bed. He worked seven days a week, excluding only his weekends "off" with the Navy Reserves.

But the hard work paid off. The company grew. Headquarters moved from the trailer to a two-story building in downtown Anaheim. Later, a branch office was established in San Diego. After that, came offices in Arizona and Nevada. Dad, who as a boy remembered going to bed hungry, had become a prosperous man. He was not one to flaunt his new wealth, however. We lived pretty much the same as we lived before. Although we could have moved to a fancier home, we stayed in the old Fullerton house. He could have bought a fancy car, but he favored a modest Pontiac convertible and his Willys Jeep. He never became a big spender.

An important family event occurred when I was twelve. Dad bought some property in Mariposa, California. Mariposa is located in the Sierra Nevada foothills about thirty miles southwest of Yosemite National Park. A friend of his from the Navy had become a real estate agent in Mariposa, and there was a 225-acre "ranch" there that had gone into foreclosure. The agent-friend called Dad and told him about the opportunity. Dad ended up buying the land strictly as an investment deal, with every intention of making a quick turnaround on the property.

However, he quickly fell in love with "the ranch." Located at an elevation of 3,200 feet, oak and pine trees grew side by side there; there was snow in the winter, and in the summer the blue-sky temperatures reached into the 90s. Two creeks flowed through the property, and there was an old, two-story farmhouse. For decades, the property had been a working ranch with crops grown in irrigated fields and cows grazing on the wild grass. At the time of foreclosure, however, the fields were unplowed, and the cows had all been sold.

The ranch quickly became the place where we now took all our summer vacations. Characteristically, my dad was not content to simply use the land as somewhere to go and relax and watch the birds. He immediately started to formulate plans for turning the property back into a working ranch. He tried his hand at chickens, geese, pheasants, emus, and honeybees. He bought a herd of twenty cows and an Angus bull with a pedigree. There were three ponds on the property, and he stocked them with trout, catfish, and bass; the ranch became a registered fishery.

My dad was now a cattle rancher and fish farmer.

*   *   *

Over the next thirty years, Dad piloted his engineering business and visited the ranch on a regular basis. However, trouble struck Willdan in the late 1990s. The company now had a board of directors, and Dad, Willdan's CEO, served "at the pleasure of" the board. Apparently, rival factions representing the two founders of the company had formed: the Stookey faction and the Walter Thein faction. Stookey and Thein now had different visions for the future of the company. In the end, the Thein faction gained the upper hand. My dad, now in his seventies, was forced to leave the company he had co-founded over three decades earlier. He would never work for Willdan or as a civil engineer again.

He did not take retirement well. Even at age seventy-five, he was still a workaholic. Work defined who he was and gave his life meaning. He could never be the type to don a Hawaiian shirt and quietly while away his "golden years" playing golf and sipping drinks topped with umbrellas and sliced fruit. Shortly after being forced out at Willdan, my dad became seriously depressed. He sat on the back porch of the house in Fullerton and for days at a time just stared out into the backyard. He was angry. He was bitter. But mostly he was lost—his reason for living had been taken away. It was strange to see my father this way, because he'd never been a depressed sort of person. He'd always had a zest for life. Now here he was, wasting away, doing nothing.

The gloom lasted about six months. My dad became so depressed that he saw a psychiatrist, and the psychiatrist put him briefly on a tranquilizer and an antidepressant. I don't know if it was the medication or simply time that effected a cure, but, eventually, my dad climbed out of his funk and found a way to get meaning back to his life. For Dad, that meaning could be found in only one place: work. He threw himself back into his ranch.

He became a cowboy. He increased the size of his herd and took on all aspects of ranch work. He would ear-tag his own cows, load his barn with bales of hay, and haul cows to auction himself pulling a cow trailer with his Jeep (he now had a new Wrangler). He redoubled his efforts as a fish farmer and began raising koi as well as trout and catfish. I don't know how much money he made with his cows and his fish (probably very little), but it didn't matter: he was working again.

38

His health remained relatively good through the next several years, but as mentioned already, it was not perfect. The heart attack at age sixty-five had made him more health conscious. He'd stopped smoking, and he was eating better. But the one health problem that would come to bother him more than anything was the knee arthritis that began to plague him as he moved into his early eighties. The problem was the arthritis had begun to limit his activities at the ranch. He tried surgery on one knee, but the disappointing result was even more knee pain than before. So, he tried everything short of further surgery (which he vowed never to consider again): Tylenol and Advil, physical therapy, glucosamine, chondroitin, even rooster comb injections and emu oil. Nothing worked. The pain got worse, and walking became more and more difficult. He hated his disability and became increasingly frustrated.

Yet, despite the knee trouble, Dad still managed to pursue most of his activities at his beloved ranch. Now he rode around the land on a motorcycle, and he managed his cattle and took an occasional cow to the auction. He continued to stock the ponds with fish. He baled hay. He laid irrigation pipe. He mended fences. He was eighty-three years old. He was happy.

Then, one night in mid-September, it all came tumbling down.

III. The Directive

When Mom and I returned to my parents' house that first night after my dad's stroke, the house seemed eerily still and quiet. I fed the cat, then micro-waved a couple of frozen dinners, and Mom poured herself a glass of wine. Sitting down at the kitchen table, we ate in silence. I should say I ate in silence; my mom hardly touched her food.

After dinner, I went to my parents' bedroom to inspect the scene. When I reached the bedroom door, I stopped and peered inside. I could see the blanket and sheet lying crumpled on the floor. One pillow was on the bed; the other was on the floor. There was blood on the carpet, a three-inch steak, on one side of the bed next to the nightstand.

Stepping into the room, I tried to piece together what might have happened during the night. My father had awoken—who knows what time?—to find himself paralyzed on the right side of his body and unable to talk. He must have struggled to get out of bed. I suspect he'd fallen to the floor, injuring himself (thus, the blood on the carpet, perhaps from a blow to the nose or mouth). Down on the floor, he struggled further, trying to stand and probably trying to alert my mother. He'd somehow dragged himself around to the foot of the bed. That was where my mom said she had found him.

Upon further inspection, I discovered something else. Lying on the floor, between the nightstand and the bed, was Dad's old Bible. That Bible was over a hundred years old, a gift handed down from his parents. For as long as I could remember, that old, tattered Bible had sat untouched on my father's nightstand, more of an heirloom than something to be opened and read.

As odd as it might sound, I really didn't know much about my father's religious views. We'd never talked much about religion in our home. He'd been raised a Baptist. There was a rumor of a grandparent who was Jewish. I knew he believed in God because he'd told me so once. However, in all my life, he'd never once gone to church. My mother, not much of a churchgoer either, had at least taken my sister and me to church on Easter Sundays when we were young—yet, even then, my father didn't go along with us. I'd always considered him to be a kind of Deist: someone who believed in God, but who had no interest in organized religion.

Nevertheless, there it lay on the floor: his old Bible. How had it gotten there? Had it accidentally fallen from the nightstand as he had struggled to get out of bed? Or, had he taken the Bible down of his own volition?

I imagined a scenario that was both touching and distressing. My father had awoken in the middle of the night half paralyzed, unable to talk or swallow. He knew something terrible had happened to his body. Somehow he managed to get from the bed to the floor, and as he lay there choking on his own saliva, he knew death was present with him in that room. Consequently, he'd dragged himself to the nightstand and pulled the Bible down.

He'd taken the book down, and he had prayed.

I cleaned up the room a little. I put the Bible back on the nightstand and put the sheet and blanket back on the bed. Using some water and hydrogen peroxide, I cleaned the bloodstain on the carpet.

Shutting the bedroom door, I went back to the kitchen to see how Mom was doing. She'd moved to the living room and was asleep on the couch. It was 8:00 PM. I took the comforter blanket that lay folded over the back of the couch, and I placed it over her. I turned off the light. Leaving her to sleep, I went to Dad's study, located at the back of the house. I knew there was a white notebook he kept there, and it contained many of his important documents. I suspected his health directive, if he had one, would be located in the notebook.

I had no trouble finding it. The notebook was sitting on the shelf above his desk. I took it down and started flipping through the pages. The notebook contained precisely the type of papers I was looking for: his Last Will and Testament, a copy of the Living Trust he'd drawn up with Mom, and…sure enough, there it was: "The Advance Health Care Directive of William C. Stookey."

The directive was six pages long. I read it from beginning to end. Most of it was boilerplate legalese with the appropriate blanks filled in. The date indicated the directive had been drawn up some ten years earlier. My mother had been designated his "health care agent" in the event of his incapacitation. I had been designated the "alternative agent" should Mom become "not available" or "ineligible to act." On page five, I found the single, all-important sentence I was looking for—the part where my father stated his wishes for hospital care in the event of serious, life-threatening illness.

"It is my desire that extra-ordinary measures not be taken to prolong my life if the result of such efforts are not likely to be successful or if the results of such efforts will not leave me in a condition where I will be able to enjoy a reasonable quality of life."

That was it, then. No "extra-ordinary measures." At first read, I took this to mean no ventilator. No chest compressions. No shocking the heart. However, as I read over that crucial sentence a second time, I started to feel a little less sure about my father's exact wishes. The language was vague and general, purposefully so, no doubt. Certain phrases like "extraordinary measures" and "reasonable quality of life" were open to interpretation. The more recent trend in advance directives was to be more specific, spelling out precise wishes regarding things like ventilators, IVs, and heart shocking. This directive had been written before that trend. Consequently, a good deal of interpretation and decision-making had been left up to my mom and me as my dad's "health care agents." It would be up to us to decode the meaning of "extra-ordinary measures" and "a reasonable quality of life."

I knew Mom would have a very hard time doing this. She had always left the hard decisions of life up to my dad, from financial investments to what model of car to drive. I knew in the matter of important life and death medical decisions, my mom would be completely overwhelmed. She was going to need help.

I read the sentence on page five a third time. "No extraordinary measures" if no "reasonable quality of life." At this point, Dad's prognosis was, to some degree, uncertain. People sometimes recover from strokes, especially mild ones. However, Dad's stroke was not a "mild one." He'd had one of the worst strokes I'd ever seen, affecting both sides of his body, his speech, and his ability to swallow. I knew the chances of his ever regaining full use of his right side were low. Realistically, I doubted he would ever walk again. I asked myself: being confined to a bed or a wheelchair, half-paralyzed, unable to talk, unable to swallow—would this be something Dad would consider "a reasonable quality of life?"

To me, the answer was obvious: of course not. Dad had always been an active, one could even say a "restless," person. He was the type of person who believed each day should be marked by the accomplishment of something productive. He disdained idleness and inactivity. There was no question in my mind—Dad would not consider his current physical state to be "a reasonable quality of life."

I knew the hospital staff would ask specifically about ventilator support and cardiac resuscitation (shocking the heart). I asked myself the question: would a ventilator somehow improve the prognosis and heal my dad's damaged brain? The answer was no. Would an electrical shock to his heart have him walking and talking again? Again, the answer was no.

I went over to the copier in the study and made a copy of the directive for the hospital. Assuming Mom agreed, I knew what we would tell the ICU staff in the morning. No ventilator. No heart shocking. No "extraordinary measures."

*   *   *

I put the white notebook back up on the shelf. I was tired. I'd been up since 5:00 AM. I went to my old bedroom and sat down on the bed. This was the house I'd grown up in, and this was the room I'd slept in till the age of eighteen. The furniture was all the same as it had been during my childhood: the single bed, the roll-top desk, the three-drawer dresser. On the dresser, Mom had long ago placed a black-and-white photo of me riding on Dad's shoulders in the yard in front of the house. I must have been three or four years old; he would have been in his early thirties. I'm wearing a train engineer's hat, and he is shirtless and muscular, wearing khaki pants. I'm holding onto his head, and we're both smiling at the camera. We look happy.

Getting into bed, I turned off the light. Sinking my head into the pillow, the vision of me sitting atop the shoulders of my young father stayed in my mind. That was so long ago, nearly fifty years. Dad was in his prime, and I was the vulnerable one. Those fifty years had passed so quickly. Where had they gone?

Lying there in my childhood bed, it was the image of my youthful, vigorous, full-of-life father that hung in my mind as I drifted off to sleep.

IV. The Neurologist

Mom and I returned to the ICU at 9:00 AM the next day. The pink-uniformed volunteer at the desk let us pass through the door. I was relieved. I feared Dad might not have made it through the night. I half-expected her to say, "Have a seat; the doctor will be out in a moment to talk to you."

We walked down the hall, again passing by the busy nursing station and the patient rooms. I had my father's advance directive in hand, inside a manila folder. I'd not yet talked to Mom about the directive. She had slept in (she said she'd woken up at 1:00 and hadn't gotten back to sleep till 5:00), and I had to wake her up in order to get to the hospital by 9:00. There hadn't been time to talk.

As we approached Bed 5, I braced myself. How would he look after a night in the intensive care unit? Better? Worse? I briefly imagined the miraculous: he would be sitting up in bed eating breakfast, like the man we'd just passed in Room 7. The first thing he would say to us would be, "Get me the hell out of here!"

However, there was no miracle. He was there, lying on his side, eyes pointed upward, his flaccid right arm propped up on a pillow. It was immediately obvious: his condition was unchanged.

We went to the side of the bed, and I took his hand. Once again, there was the flicker of recognition on his face when he saw me. "Hey, how are you doing?" I said.

My dad made a weak attempt to say something, a slight movement of his mouth without sound. He seemed weaker. Yesterday, at least, he'd made garbled noises when he tried to speak. Today there was no sound at all, just the weak movement of the mouth. I pressed my fingers into the palm of his right hand. "Squeeze," I said. "Squeeze my fingers." I was looking to see if he was getting any strength back on the right side. "Squeeze!"

The hand was lifeless. Dead weight. No change. I stepped back and made room for Mom.

"Hi, Bill," she said. "Hi, Honey." I could see my mom, too, was looking for signs of improvement. "Are you feeling better?"

While she talked, I checked Dad's vital signs displayed on the monitor above the bed. His vitals remained stable: pulse, blood pressure, oxygen level. Looking back at him, I made an accounting of all the tubes and probes attached to his body: heart electrodes, oxygen tubing, IV in the right forearm, blood pressure cuff on the left arm, Foley (urine) catheter, pneumatic stockings (leg stockings that inflated and deflated in order to prevent blood clots in the calves).

I looked around the room. The wall-mounted television displayed a bucolic mountain scene with pine trees, green meadows, and a running stream. A soothing flute melody played over the audio. The intent was obviously to soothe the occupant of the room, and I thought it was a nice touch. The mountain scene was reminiscent of Dad's ranch. *Good*, I thought. He would like that.

Just then, two women walked briskly into room—a middle-aged woman wearing a blue blouse and a younger woman wearing black scrubs. "Hello-o-o," the woman in the blouse said cheerily. "Is this Mr. Stookey?" she asked, looking at Dad. Of course, he didn't respond.

"Yes," I said. "I'm Chris, his son, and this is Betty, his wife."

"Hi, we're from speech therapy," the woman in the

blouse said. "The doctor has ordered a swallowing test for Mr. Stookey."

"A what?" Mom asked.

"Swallowing test. We want to see how well Mr. Stookey—Bill—can swallow. If he passes the test, he'll be able to start eating something today. You'd like that, wouldn't you Bill? Huh?" The woman put her hand on Dad's shoulder and smiled broadly. He made a movement with his mouth that looked almost like an attempt to say, "Yes." It occurred to me that he probably *was* hungry—he'd had nothing to eat in over twenty-four hours.

The younger woman in the scrubs had a brown paper bag in her hand. She pulled a table on wheels over to the bedside and put the bag on it. The connection between speech therapy and swallowing might not seem immediately obvious. However, I knew this was the tradition in most hospitals: speech therapy does the swallowing testing on stroke patients.

"How is Bill doing today, Mrs. Stookey?" the woman in the blouse asked. She was obviously the one in charge. She did all the talking.

"Well," Mom said, "we just got here. Are you the doctor?"

"No. I'm the speech therapist."

The woman in the scrubs put on some plastic gloves and set up the suction device at the head of my dad's bed. She turned on the suction and tucked the suction catheter under Dad's pillow.

"Okay, let's go!" the woman in the blouse said, opening up the brown bag. She took out a cup of ice cream, a cup of pudding, and a cup of apple sauce. "We always start with the ice cream," she said. "If he passes that, we move on to the pudding. Now, the first thing I'm going to do is put the head of the bed up a little more." Using the electronic controls, she raised up the head of Dad's bed. He grimaced as his head rose, the left corner of his mouth pulling down as though the sudden movement had caused some pain. As his head rose further, he began to side off his pillows; his body slumped to the right and pressed up against the bed rails.

"Whoops!" the woman said. Her helper repositioned my dad so he was straight and upright.

"That's better," the woman in the blouse said as she stripped off the top of the ice cream cup. "Now, Bill, what I'm going to do is put a small bit of ice cream in your mouth. Actually, it's not ice cream. It's sherbet. Raspberry."

"He's a little hard of hearing," Mom said.

"Oh, sorry!" the woman said. She leaned down and spoke loudly next to my dad's ear. "I'm going to give you some sherbet, Bill, and we'll see how well you can swallow it. Okay?"

Dad made a noise, like a grunt. I was surprised. Suddenly, he seemed more alert and interactive than when we'd first arrived. He seemed to understand what was going on.

The woman in the blouse took out a plastic spoon and scooped up a quarter spoon-full of sherbet. "O-ka-a-a-y!" She held the spoon up. "Yum!" She put the spoon to Dad's lips, and he immediately sucked the sherbet off the spoon. He made some smacking motions with his lips, and you could see he was manipulating the sherbet in his mouth as it melted. "Good!" the woman said, "There you go." She turned to Mom and me and smiled. "He's taking it, see?"

We stood and watched. A small bit of the red goo began to drip down the right corner of Dad's mouth. "Oops!" the woman said. She grabbed a napkin and daubed up the sherbet. Nevertheless, she turned back to us and smiled again. It appeared he might pass the sherbet test.

Then, suddenly, he began to cough. A little choking at first, then a full cough. The first cough was followed by a second stronger cough, and he coughed the sherbet onto his chin and chest. Then he took a breath and immediately coughed again—much worse this time. He coughed so hard his face turned red. Not good. More coughing.

"Suction!" the woman in the blouse ordered.

The woman in the scrubs hurried to place the plastic suction catheter into my Dad's mouth, and she suctioned out the gooey, pink saliva. After the suctioning, he stopped coughing.

The woman in the blouse silently cleaned my father's chin and mouth with a napkin. There was a solemn frown on her face. Her cheeriness was suddenly gone. "Unfortunately," she said slowly, "that's an obvious fail. He's lost his swallowing reflex. Not what we wanted. If we feed him by mouth, he'll aspirate and choke." She looked at my mom and shook her head. "Sorry."

"He can't have any more?" Mom asked.

"No, not by mouth." The woman picked up the cup of sherbet and put it in a plastic bag. "He'll probably need a feeding tube," she said tying a knot in the bag. "Of course, that'll be up to the doctor. I'll let him know the results of the test."

The woman in the scrubs turned off the suction. She removed her gloves and tossed them in the trash, and she placed the pudding and the applesauce back in the paper bag.

"What's a feeding tube?" Mom asked.

The woman in the blouse lowered Dad's head back down. "It's a tube that…. The doctor will explain it. He'll go over everything. I'll call him right now and let him know." She made a small apologetic bow and joined her assistant, who was at the door. She and her assistant left the room and hurried down the corridor.

Mom looked at me with a worried look on her face. "What's a feeding tube?" she asked again.

"It goes in the nose and into the stomach," I said. "For feeding, because he can't swallow."

"In the nose?"

"Yeah. Nose, down the throat."

The worry lines on Mom's face deepened further. 'Oh," was all she said.

"They can also do an operation where they put the tube directly into the stomach, here," I said pointing to my own stomach. "It'd be better if he could swallow on his own, obviously. But, if he tries to eat…. You saw what happened. If food gets into his lungs, he'll get pneumonia—that's bad."

"Pneumonia?"

"Yes."

My mom turned to Dad and took his hand. The ordeal with the sherbet seemed to have tired him out—there were no longer any signs of expression on the good side his face. He seemed to be breathing a little fast, as well. I looked at the heart monitor. His pulse was up.

"Why are his eyes that way?" Mom asked after a moment. I don't know if it was the first time she'd noticed his leftward gaze or if she'd only just now summoned up the courage to ask about it.

"It's part of the stroke," I said. "It affected the part of his brain that controls the eyes."

I pulled a chair over to the side of the bed for my mom. Sitting in the chair, she went silent. She held Dad's hand and gently stroked it. But she said nothing more.

Half an hour later, the neurologist arrived. He was a

tallish man, in his mid-forties, thin to the point of being gaunt, wearing a cream shirt and blue tie but no white coat. He introduced himself as Dr. Alexander. I identified Mom and myself and offered a handshake (otherwise, he would not have bothered).

"You're a physician," Alexander said. "Emergency?"

"Yes." I recalled the nurse from yesterday who said "the neurologist" had seen my dad in the ER; I guessed the ER physician had told Alexander that Mr. Stookey had a physician son.

Having identified me as a physician, Alexander spoke almost exclusively to me, largely ignoring Mom. He used "doctor's language" and employed words and terms I knew were completely foreign to her. It was as though she didn't exist. His manner was confident but dry as desert sand.

"So, your father's had a significant insult," he said. "The MRI shows a large area of ischemic infarction on the left side of the brain."

"You did an MRI?" I asked.

"Yes, last night. It shows there's also some right-brain involvement. So, probably multiple cardiac emboli."

Translation: your father had a large stroke, as confirmed by an MRI scan. The scan shows parts of both the right side and the left side of the brain have been affected. The cause of the stroke is likely multiple blood clots that formed in your dad's heart, broke away, and traveled to his brain. The clots then acted like plugs that cut off the blood flow to large areas of the brain.

"The MRI shows the area of speech comprehension is spared," Alexander said. "So, your father has an expressive aphasia, but his speech comprehension is probably intact."

Translation: although your dad cannot talk to us, he likely

52

understands what we are saying to him. This made sense, I thought. It would explain my dad's facial expressions. He couldn't speak because the part of the brain controlling the *muscles* of speech had been affected. But he could understand.

My first thought was the sparing of the speech area was a good thing. However, on second thought, I wasn't so sure. This meant Dad was probably more fully conscious than he appeared to be. He could think and form language in his mind, and he could understand other people speaking. Yet he could not speak or express himself. It was like being trapped inside one's own body.

Alexander now went about performing a physical exam on Dad. He shined a light in my dad's eyes, checked his limb strength and muscle tone, and listened to his heart and lungs with his stethoscope. He spoke to me while doing the exam. "So, as I'm sure you've noticed, your father is unable to swallow. He's at a very high risk for aspiration. A chest x-ray done this morning already shows early signs of bilateral pneumonia. That's why we've started the antibiotics."

Alexander gestured toward the IV pole above Dad's bed. I hadn't noticed it before, but there was now a bag containing an antibiotic dripping into the IV. "He failed his swallowing test this morning. So, he's going to need an NG tube for feedings. I looked through the chart, and there's no advance directive."

"I have it here," I said. I picked up the manila folder, opened it, and handed the directive to Alexander. "It doesn't say anything specifically about feeding tubes."

Alexander took the directive and quickly glanced through it. "So…."

He said "so" a lot.

"So, do you know your father's wishes regarding

ventilator support and cardiac resuscitation?" he asked.

For the first time, he looked at Mom. He'd obviously seen that *she* was my dad's primary "health care agent." She had been listening intently, but she had no idea what we were talking about.

"He doesn't want extraordinary measures," I said to Alexander.

"So, no heart shocking or respirator?" Alexander asked.

I turned to Mom. "That paper, the advance directive, Dad wrote it. It says…." I paused and turned back toward Alexander. "Can we step outside for a minute?" I asked. Since my dad might understand what we were saying, I thought it would be better to have this discussion outside the room.

All three of us stepped outside.

"The directive," I said to Mom, standing in the hall, "it says he doesn't want any extraordinary measures. That means things like putting him on a breathing machine and having his heart shocked. Did he ever talk to you about this stuff?"

"No," Mom said. She suddenly looked very scared.

"I don't think he'd want the breathing machine," I said to Mom. "It would be like his mother."

Mom understood the reference to Dad's mother and her protracted, painful death.

"Let me be frank," Alexander said. "The MRI shows extensive areas of brain loss. So, he's not going to regain function in those areas. Does that mean there's no chance of any improvement? No. With extensive physical therapy, some people retrain other parts of the brain and get some function back. But I will be honest with you: there's not a lot of motor cortex left for retraining. So, in my opinion, the best you can expect is some minimal improvement. If that."

Mom stared at me in silence. A tear slid down her cheek.

"His mom died of cancer," I explained to Alexander. "It was... a slow process. He didn't want—to be like that."

"So, that's a no on the respirator and heart shocks? Mrs. Stookey?"

My mom grabbed my hand. I think she did it because she needed support standing up. "Whatever Chris wants," she said, her voice barely audible.

"No on the respirator and no on the heart shocks," I said solemnly to Alexander.

"What about a feeding tube?" he asked, again addressing Mom.

Mom looked at me.

"Remember, he can't eat," I said. "He can't swallow."

"My recommendation," Alexander said, "is we go ahead with the tube for now. In general, a feeding tube is not considered an extraordinary measure. We can work with speech and physical therapy and see if the swallowing improves, see if the feeding tube can be removed at a later time."

"He needs to eat," Mom said.

"Okay," I said. "We'll do the feeding tube."

"Very well," Alexander said. He glanced at his watch. "I'll write the order for a nasogastric tube, and I'll put the advance directive in the chart indicating no respirator and no cardiac resuscitation. Agreed?"

I nodded my head. Agreed.

Alexander stuffed his stethoscope into his pants pocket. "So, I'm going to do another MRI today," he said. "I think his condition might have deteriorated somewhat during the night. He seems weaker today. I want to see if there's been an extension of his stroke or perhaps some hemorrhage. They'll take him later this morning. I'll order the MRI now."

Alexander turned on his heels and, without saying goodbye, walked away.

I didn't like him much. I'm sure he was a perfectly competent neurologist. I had no disagreement with his diagnosis or even his pronouncement of the grim prognosis. But he'd been frosty cold in delivering the bleak news. And I didn't like the way he spoke to me in medicalese, while ignoring my mom. He could have least offered his condolences to her in plain English.

Mom and I started back into my dad's room. But as we stepped through the door, my mom tugged my sleeve and stopped me. She looked down the hallway where Alexander had disappeared. Then, looking back at me, she said:

"Just so I understand…."

"Understand what, Mom?"

"That man…."

"Yes?"

"Was he the doctor?"

*   *   *

When they took Dad away for the second MRI, Mom and I went back to the Fullerton house for lunch.

As we left the room, we ran into one of the floor janitors who was mopping the hall. She was a short, late-middle-aged woman, Hispanic, wearing gray overalls. Upon seeing us, the woman stopped her mopping. She stepped aside and gave us a smile.

"Oh, don't you look pretty in your red sweater!" she said sweetly to my mom. There was genuineness in her voice, and a look of kindness in her eyes.

"Thank you," my mom said, brightening.

"Watch your step, now," the woman said. "Wet floor." She looked at me and smiled. From the sympathetic look on her face, I could tell she understood our situation, and she had tried to say something positive to us, something to cheer my mom a little. It was a small thing, but it meant a lot at that moment. A small bit of human warmth reaching out, if only for a brief touch.

I turned around as we went down the hall and looked back at the woman, who was standing with her mop looking back at us. She smiled at me again and gave a little wave.

I smiled back and mouthed: *Thank you.*

*   *   *

Lori joined us when we returned to the hospital that afternoon. She'd taken the afternoon off work so she could visit Dad. She drove up to the Fullerton house just as Mom and I were coming out. We got into Lori's car, and the three of us drove back to St. Mark's.

"He's pretty bad," I said to Lori. "I just want to prepare you for that. He can't talk, and he can't swallow." I told Lori about our decision to place the feeding tube. She agreed it was the right thing to do.

The first thing I noticed when we arrived to Room 5 was there was an NG tube sticking out of my dad's nose. They'd wasted no time putting it in. There was a large bottle of vanilla-milkshake-like feeding solution hanging from the IV pole above his bed. The solution dripped slowly into the feeding tube. I stepped up to the side of the bed. Dad's eyes were open.

"Lori's here," I said. I stepped back and allowed Lori to take my place at the bedside. "Take his left hand," I said.

"That's his good side. He knows you're there, and he feels you touch him."

"Hi," Lori said, taking his hand. It was all she could say, and it came out almost in a whisper. Lori stared down at Dad in silence. Even though I'd tried to prepare her, I think the reality of his condition was beyond what she had expected.

He seemed to recognize her. He moved his lips when she took his hand, as though trying to say something.

"They put the feeding tube in," I said to my mom. "See?"

Mom looked at the tube and followed it up to the bottle of feeding solution. "What's in the bottle?" she asked.

"Feeding solution," I said. "You know, proteins, sugars, vitamins. Like a milkshake."

Mom nodded her approval at the word "vitamins." "Good," she said. "That's what he needs."

I got chairs for my mom and my sister, and they sat at the bedside. There were only two chairs in the room, so I leaned against the sink counter. I watched while they sat talking to Dad, carrying on a one-sided conversation. Occasionally, he would cough a little. Mom, by now used to this, calmly wiped the saliva away with a Kleenex.

We stayed until they closed down for visiting hours at 6:00. During that time, the icy ICU nurse and an attendant came into the room every couple hours to turn my dad from side to side. I asked the nurse about the second MRI. She said it had been done, but she didn't know the results.

On the drive home, my sister asked the obvious question. "Is he going to get better?"

"I don't know," I said. "He doesn't seem any better today—I mean, compared to yesterday."

"He's really bad," Lori said.

"I know," I said. "The neurologist thinks…. Well, he said

58

the prognosis isn't good. He doesn't know if there'll be a lot of improvement. If any."

"There's nothing they can do?" Lori asked.

"No, that's the thing with strokes. There's no operation; there's no magic pill."

"So it's just a matter of wait and see?"

"Yeah," I said. "Pretty much."

As my sister and I talked, Mom, still wearing her "pretty" red sweater and holding her purse in her lap, stared silently out the passenger's window at the passing traffic.

V. Hemlock

When Mom and I arrived the next morning, Dr. Alexander was already in Room 5 examining Dad, checking his reflexes with a reflex hammer.

"How's he doing?" I asked.

"Same," Alexander said dryly, as he continued his reflex check.

"What about the MRI?" I asked.

"There could be some increased subtle swelling of the brain due to the stroke. Otherwise, unchanged." Alexander put his reflex hammer in his pants pocket and turned toward me. "It's been over forty-eight hours now," he said, "and we're not seeing any improvement. The chances of there being any significant improvement going forward are not good."

Mom's shoulders dropped. I put my arm around her.

"I see," I said.

"I'm going to order a CAT scan."

Why? I wondered. What for? Another test? What difference would it make?

"I want to be sure there's no post-stroke bleeding of the brain," Alexander said as if he'd read my mind. "It's unlikely, but I want to be sure. If the CAT scan doesn't show anything new, we'll transfer him out of the ICU this afternoon or tomorrow. There's not much more we can do for him here in intensive care."

I squeezed Mom's shoulder. "All right," I said. Alexander was already backing out of the door. He seemed to be in a hurry. But, really, what else was there for him to say? His bedside manner was terrible, but, at least, he'd been honest. He scuttled out the door and hurried down the hall.

I looked at Mom. There were tears in her eyes. The neurologist, the brain specialist, had just told us Dad's dismal condition was probably not going to improve. My mom hadn't understood the medical jargon, but the look on her face indicated she'd understood at least this much: *Chance of improvement not good. Nothing we can do.*

I went to the bedside and took hold of Dad's left hand. His eyes were closed, but he opened them when I took his hand. He moved his left toes a bit and squeezed back with his hand—weakly, but a squeeze, nonetheless. He knew I was there. Had he, too, heard Dr. Alexander's grim prognosis?

"Hi," I said. "Were you sleeping?"

He closed his eyes.

I moved aside and let Mom take my place. I brought over a chair, and she sat down. "Are you warm enough, Bill?" she asked with a slight tremor in her voice. "You just have one sheet." Dad opened his eyes again as my mom spoke. She stood up and pulled the blanket up, folding it down at Dad's chest. Taking hold of his hand, she sat back down.

We sat in silence. The TV was off, and the only sound in the room was the sound of the pump working to move feeding fluid through the NG tube.

Sitting there at the bedside, I thought about what lay ahead. My father was never going to walk again. He was probably never going to talk again. He was probably never going to take food or even water by mouth again. Soon they would move him out of the ICU to a regular hospital bed. Then what?

He couldn't stay in the hospital forever. Would we take him home? How would we feed him? Would he need an operation to place a permanent feeding tube (the one in his nose was temporary)? How would we bathe him? Handle his

61

bathroom needs? But if we couldn't handle this at home, what then? A nursing home? The idea made me cringe. My father would never, never in a thousand years, want to be in a nursing home. Although he had never told me this directly, I knew it with absolute certainty. To Dad, it would be worse than being imprisoned. But, what other options did we have?

We stayed with him for another two hours. He drifted in and out of sleep. The now-familiar ICU nurse came in to hang a fresh dose of IV antibiotics. She came back a little later to empty out the urine in his Foley catheter bag. Then, at 11:00, a transportation tech came in to take him away for the CAT scan.

Mom kissed him goodbye. We watched as the tech wheeled him out the door and down the hall. It was so strange to see Dad so completely at the mercy of others, lying passively in bed, being wheeled away by a stranger for another medical test. Had anyone asked *him* if he wanted another CAT scan? Had anyone asked him if he wanted any of this? The NG tube, the IV in his arm, the Foley catheter, more tests? I suspected he didn't want any of it.

I recalled how Mom had said Dad didn't want the paramedics to take him to the hospital. "'No, no,'" Mom had said. "He kept saying, 'No, no.'"

The tech rolled Dad into an elevator, and the door shut. Mom and I headed home for lunch.

*   *   *

That afternoon, I began going through some of my father's mail. I sat down at his study desk and began opening envelopes. There were bank statements and utility bills, along with the usual junk mail. Everything was in his name; he took care of all financial matters. Mom had her own small bank account, used mainly for buying groceries and household items. Was she also a signatory on the main account? Should I contact the bank and tell them about what had happened? Had my dad made any sort of financial arrangements in the case of his incapacitation?

I turned again to the white notebook to see if it contained any answers. I read through the trust document, "The William and Betty Stookey Trust." The trust contained a lot of dense legalese, but I was able to decipher the important parts: the bank accounts, stock portfolios, and property holdings were all held jointly in the trust by my dad *and* my mom.

This came as a relief. It meant Mom had access to all the accounts. I could help her with the household bills and finances—all she had to do was sign the checks. I would later discover that Mom was only vaguely aware of the existence of the trust. She recalled that, some years ago, Dad had asked her to sign some documents, and she'd dutifully done so without really knowing what it was she was signing. No matter, though, the trust was there, and the bank accounts were held jointly.

In addition to the white notebook, I knew Dad kept a lot of his other important papers in his desk drawer. Going through the drawer, there were about two-dozen labeled files inside. I read the various file names: "Mariposa Cattle," "Bank Statements," "Social Security." There was a file for his health insurance. That was an important file, and I took it out and went through it. Funny, I thought. No one at the hospital had asked us about Dad's insurance status. There was no doubt in my mind the hospital had already looked into this. I knew that the paramedics often picked up identification and health insurance cards when they took a patient to the hospital. Fortunately, Dad was fully insured by both Medicare and

Tricare, the military retiree health benefits program. I left the health file out, thinking I might bring it to the hospital.

I continued going through the drawer. There was a file relating to my dad's plan to donate money to The Desert Tortoise Club of California. I smiled when I saw this. Dad had developed a fondness for desert tortoises when he'd encountered them doing some engineering work in the Mohave Desert years ago. It saddened him that the tortoises were a threatened species. He even kept two desert tortoises in his backyard at home, a male and a female.

The last file I found turned out to be something quite important and highly pertinent to my dad's current situation. It was not something I was looking for or anything I'd expected to find. The file was labeled simply, and somewhat cryptically, "Hemlock."

I immediately suspected this might be something important. "Hemlock," of course, is a poisonous plant, and Socrates, the Greek philosopher, famously drank hemlock tea in an act of suicide. I tried to remember: Wasn't there a "right-to-die" group called the "Hemlock Society?"

I took "Hemlock" out of the drawer and opened the folder. There was not a lot inside, just three items. The first item was an issue of *Time* magazine dated September 18, 2000. The picture on the cover was a black-and-white face shot of a gray-bearded man with oxygen tubing in his nostrils; his mouth was open, his head back, his eyes closed. It was, quite obviously, the picture of a man on the cusp of death.

The title on the magazine cover was, "Dying On Our Own Terms." The caption beneath the title read: *"Too many Americans spend their final days in a hospital or nursing home, alone and in pain. It doesn't have to be that way."* My heart began to race a little. This all seemed so pertinent to the questions I'd been asking myself a short time ago in the ICU, questions about what lay ahead for my dad. I opened the magazine to the feature article, "A Kinder, Gentler Death" and read the opening lines. "Dying is one of the few events in life certain to occur—and yet one we are not likely to plan for. We will spend more time getting ready for two weeks away from work than we will for our last two weeks on earth. As Moliere joked, 'We die only once—and for so long!'"

I skimmed through the article. It was full of statistics such as: "Seven out of ten Americans say they want to die at home; instead, three-fourths die in medical institutions. More than a third of dying people spend at least ten days in intensive-care units where they often endure tortuous (generally futile) attempts at a cure." A significant part of the article was devoted to the issue of pain and how doctors could do a better job of controlling it in dying patients. Another large part focused on explaining the option of hospice care, i.e., end of life care that emphasizes comfort over cure.

The article told the story of "John," an eighty-year-old man who had colon cancer and had chosen hospice after surgery had failed to achieve a cure. John and his family spoke favorably of hospice. "Nine days in the hospital [for surgery] was more than enough," John said. "Now I am home, enjoying the life I have."

I closed the magazine. How was I to interpret this? Was this my dad, his voice now cut off by the stroke, speaking to me through the article?

The second item in "Hemlock" was a ten-page pamphlet produced by "The Death With Dignity Alliance." According to the cover page, the alliance was made up of medical, legal, and academic professionals advocating "for the right of terminally-ill Americans to choose not to endure unnecessary suffering at the end of life." Leafing through the pamphlet, I saw it echoed much of what had been said in the *Time* article. It contained information on hospice care, and it, too, emphasized the importance of controlling pain in terminally ill patients.

However, the pamphlet went further. More so than the *Time* essay, the pamphlet discussed strategies to hasten death in situations of terminal illness. There was a section on a patient's right to stop all medical therapy, including refusing breathing machines, all tubes, and the taking of life-sustaining medications. There was a section on how a patient might choose to stop eating and drinking and to refuse all fluids and nutrition. There was a section on "physician-assisted death" (the alliance clearly supported the Oregon Death with Dignity Act). The final section in the pamphlet was labeled "Self-administration of Life-ending Medication," and someone—presumably my father—had placed a pencil check mark next to the first sentence of this section. Verbatim, the sentence read as follows:

> "Members of the Death with Dignity Alliance advocate a reform in the law to allow a mentally-competent, terminally ill adult to receive a prescription for a medication that may be taken at a time of the patient's own choosing, to assist a prolonged and difficult dying process."

It was pretty clear by now why the folder was called "Hemlock." I recalled the words Dad had said to me years ago, referring to his own father's suicide: "I don't blame my father for what he did. Given what Mom went through, I would do the same thing." I set down the pamphlet and leaned back in my chair. I asked myself again: Was this file a message from my father? "*In case something happens to me, please read this material—these are my wishes.*" Was "Hemlock" Dad's way of letting us know what he had not been able to tell us directly? Had my father made up the folder both for himself *and* for us?

The final item in the folder had nothing to do with hospice care or physician-assisted death or suicide. It was the Winter 2005 issue of the *Navy Retirees' Newsletter.* The *Newsletter* was folded open to page nine, to an article titled "Burial at Sea Program US Navy Mortuary Affairs." The article described a Navy program whereby any former member of the US Navy could opt to have his remains buried at sea. Family members could turn over the remains of a loved one, either "cremated or casketed," to the commander of a US Navy vessel about to deploy. During the deployment, the remains would receive an ocean burial, and the commanding officer would record the time, longitude, and latitude of the event. This information would be transmitted to the family. The article gave the names and phone numbers of contact officials.

Another message from my father? *These are my wishes for burial.* He'd been quite thorough. He'd thought of everything. I closed the folder. I knew all this was something I would have to talk about with my mom and my sister. I toyed with the idea of showing it to Mom now. She was in the living room taking a nap on the sofa. I decided, however, now was not the time. It was too soon. Not while Dad was still in intensive care. There was still a chance that he might start to show some improvement. It was too early to give up hope. I put "Hemlock" back in the file rack and closed the desk drawer.

*　　*　　*

When Mom and I returned to the hospital that afternoon,

the volunteer at the ICU desk told us Dad had been moved to a regular medical bed on the first floor.

We rode the elevator downstairs in silence. We found him in Room 23. It was a shared room, but the other bed in the room was not occupied. Dad was in the bed nearest the door, head propped up, lying on his side, looking as he'd looked in the ICU but without all the monitoring equipment. He was awake and moving his left arm a little.

We went to the bedside and said hello. I did my own mini-neurological exam, testing my dad's strength and speech. He was unchanged. No better—or worse—than he'd been in the ICU. We sat with him and talked to him. I turned on the TV. We watched part of a movie. Dad fell asleep.

At 3:00 PM, a tall woman in her thirties stepped into the room. She was wearing a tan dress and a white medical coat. She said she was a social worker, and she had been assigned to my dad's case. Looking at me, she asked if I was Chris, Mr. Stookey's son. I answered in the affirmative, and she asked if she could talk to me for a minute. Her manner was brusque and business-like—she rather reminded me of Dr. Alexander. She turned toward the door indicating, without explanation or apology to Mom, that she wanted to speak to me in private.

I followed her across the hall to the nursing station, and we stood at the counter.

"My understanding is your dad has had a very serious stroke," she said. "You're a doctor?"

"Yes."

"I spoke with Dr. Alexander. He indicated your father is likely going to need fulltime assistance for the foreseeable future. Have you thought about what you're going to do when your father leaves the hospital?"

"Well, I know my dad would prefer to be home."

68

The woman frowned. "Yes, of course. But, my understanding is your father's going to require tube feedings, bathings, catheter care, skin care, turning to prevent bedsores. It's a big job. Frankly, Chris, I know from experience it's more than most families can handle at home. Have you thought about a nursing home? I think it might be a more practical way to go."

Before I could express my thoughts, the social worker launched into what was obviously her well-rehearsed nursing home speech.

"Now. I have a list of all the nursing homes in your area." She handed me a multi-page list. "I recommend you visit at least three homes before making a final choice. The cost of each is listed. Medicare covers the entire cost for the first twenty days; then it's co-pay for the next eighty days; after that you're on your own. However, financial assistance is often available."

"My father doesn't want to go to a nursing home," I said, interrupting her momentum.

"But is bringing him home realistic, Chris? I mean, we're looking at diaper changes, Foley catheter care. He needs to be repositioned every two hours to prevent bedsores, and that alone takes two people. You could hire an attendant. But this will be a round-the-clock job, three hundred and sixty-five days a year. No breaks, no holidays, no days off. How old is your mother?"

"Eighty-three."

"Is *she* up to the task? It's just that I've seen it so many times: people take a family member home only to realize they're in over their heads."

"I understand. It's just something my dad never wanted."

"No one envisions themselves living in a nursing home.

69

But then things happen, and suddenly there aren't a lot of options."

"My dad felt strongly about it."

"Well then." The social worker let out a sigh. It was plain to see she was unhappy with my reluctance. "I can help you find home attendants, if that's what you decide. But, honestly, you should at least check a few of these homes. Some are really quite nice. _Quite_ nice. Many have twenty-four-hour-a-day visiting hours. You could visit your dad as often as you like."

I said I would discuss the matter with my mom. Along with the list of nursing homes, the social worker gave me a pamphlet titled, "Choosing the Right Nursing Home for Your Loved One." I thanked her.

"I'll talk to you tomorrow for an update?" the social worker said.

"Yes," I said. "Sure."

I went back to my dad's room. Mom was still sitting in a chair next to the bed, holding Dad's hand. "Who was that?" she asked.

"Social worker."

"Social worker?"

I looked at Dad. His eyes were closed, and he was breathing heavily. He was asleep. I lowered my voice. "She wants to know if we would consider moving Dad to a nursing home."

"A nursing home?" Mom said. The perpetual worry-wrinkle in her brow deepened. "No. I don't want him going to a nursing home."

"Yeah," I said. "Me neither."

"Your father wouldn't want that."

"I know," I said. "They just want us to start thinking about what we're going to do when he leaves the hospital."

70

"He needs to get better first."

"But, Mom…there's not a lot more they can do for him in the hospital."

"We'll take him home, then."

"Yeah, I agree. But it's not that simple. He's going to require a lot of care. The feeding tube. Bathing. How does he go to the bathroom?"

"We'll manage," Mom said.

I looked at Dad sleeping, breathing heavily, the side of his face drooping, a thin line of saliva trickling down from the corner of his mouth. "Mom," I said, "you need to understand: he might not get better. I wish I could say he would, but this is a bad stroke. He might not get any better at all. That's what the neurologist said."

"I don't want him in any nursing home."

"I agree with that. But we need to think about how much work bringing him home is going to be. I won't be able to stay with you all the time. I have to get back to work. We'll probably have to hire a nurse or someone to help."

Mom fell silent. Her lower lip trembled. I put my arm around her, and we sat together in silence. Enough, I thought. Enough for now.

VI. The Family Doctor

We stayed with Dad until dinnertime, then went home. I heated a couple more frozen dinners in the microwave. Mom didn't eat much, as usual. She went into the living room and turned on the TV.

At 7:00 PM, the phone rang. I went into the kitchen and answered.

"Hi, Chris. This is John Wilber."

"Yes?" I said. I wasn't sure who John Wilber was.

"Your dad's doctor."

"Oh, yes," I said. "Hi." Now I remembered. Dr. Wilber, the family medicine physician; he'd been my dad's primary doc for over ten years. I'd never met or talked with him before.

"How are you doing, Chris?" His voice was kind and unhurried.

"Oh … I'm okay," I said.

"Yes, of course." There was a pause. Then Wilber said: "Now, Chris, tell me, how are you *really* doing?"

The question—and its sincerity—took me by surprise. I suppose I'd gotten used to the more "concise" styles of Dr. Alexander, the social worker, and the ICU nurse.

"The stroke, it's been rough," I said. "I won't deny it. It's hard to see my dad that way, paralyzed, unable to talk, completely helpless. My dad was always the strong one of the family, and now he's completely helpless. There's a void at the top of the family structure, and there're some hard decisions to make. To be perfectly honest, it's all a bit overwhelming."

Wilber said my feelings were completely justified, and he understood why I would be feeling overwhelmed. "I guess

72

you're the one filling that void at the top now. Aren't you, Chris?"

"Yeah," I said. "I guess so."

"How about your mom? How's she holding up?" Wilber was my mom's primary physician, too, and he knew her well.

I said she was hanging in there, but just barely.

"She's lucky to have you," Wilber said. "I can't imagine how she could cope with this on her own."

Wilber then went into a layman's update on my dad's status. He knew I was a doctor; nevertheless, he spoke to me using simple terms, without a lot of medical jargon, as though this were his habit. He'd been to the hospital twice to see my dad, and he'd talked to Dr. Alexander. The MRI showed the damage was extensive.

"I know it's hard, but I don't think your dad is going to get much better," he said solemnly.

"I know," I said. "Dr. Alexander said as much. I spoke with the social worker today. She wants us to start looking at nursing homes."

There was another pause. Then Wilber said, "Tell me, Chris. How do you think your father would feel about that?"

"About going to a nursing home?"

"Uh huh."

"I don't think he would like the idea."

"I think you're right. In fact, I know you are. Your dad and I talked about it in my office, many times. We talked about a lot of things, and I've gotten to know your dad pretty well. You know what he likes to talk about more than anything?"

"What?"

"His ranch."

"Yeah. Sounds like him."

"Yup. Mariposa. He loves to talk about how much fun he

73

has chasing his cows around up there. You can see his eyes light up when he talks about his farm. He loves that place."

"I know," I said.

"About five years ago, your dad started to get arthritis in his knees. You know about that, I'm sure. He couldn't be as active at the ranch anymore. That really got him down, and we had some frank discussions about his wishes were he ever to become more severely disabled."

Wilber paused. Then he went on.

"Your dad once said to me, and to the best of my recollection this is an exact quote, 'If I ever get to the point where I can't go to the ranch and chase my cows—well, life at that point wouldn't be worth living.' Does that ring true to you, Chris? Can you hear your dad saying that?"

"Yes, actually. I can."

"You know your dad better than I do, of course. He told me you visit the house in Fullerton quite often. He's quite proud of you, you know. He loves you very much. But you know that."

"Yes. I know."

Wilber's tone became suddenly more somber. "Chris, I'm certain your dad would never want to go to a nursing home. I know that because he told me so."

"I'm not disagreeing," I said. "I don't want him to go to a nursing home either. I'm just saying that's what the social worker suggested. She felt bringing him home would be a lot of work."

"Chris, I'd like to set up a family meeting. Tomorrow, if we can. I'm free in the afternoon. Can we meet at the hospital? I'd like for us to visit together with your dad. Then we'll go sit down and talk in the family conference room. I'd like everyone to be there: you, your mom, and your sister."

74

"I'll need to talk to my sister, but I think I can arrange it."

"Two o'clock?"

"All right."

"This is something the whole family needs to be together on. You see, Chris, I'm going to advocate you don't put your dad in any nursing home."

"I'm good with that," I said.

"Your dad wants to come home, and that's what I'm going to say tomorrow. I also want to talk about his care at home. That feeding tube, for example. I want to talk about that."

"You know, he can't swallow," I said. "They did a swallowing test. He failed."

"I know."

Another long pause.

"You don't think my dad wants the feeding tube, do you?" I asked.

"That's one of the things I want to talk about tomorrow," Wilber said.

It wasn't hard to read between the lines. Of course, if we stopped the tube feeds, my dad would die. It was that simple. I replayed what Wilber had just said my dad had told him: *If I ever get to the point where I can't go to the ranch and chase my cows— well, life at that point wouldn't be worth living.*

"It's a conversation we need to have," Wilber said.

"That's going to be a hard conversation for my mom." It was all I could say.

"I know. Your mom and I go way back."

"She still hopes he'll get better."

"Of course she does," Wilber said. "That's exactly what we need to talk about. Two o'clock? In your dad's room at the hospital?"

I had moved into Dad's study as Wilber and I talked. I stood now at the window looking out into the backyard. Under the yard lights, I could see the water running down the fountain of the koi pond—the koi pond my dad had built more than thirty years ago.

"All right," I said. "Two o'clock."

*   *   *

After the phone call with Wilber, I went out into the backyard. I stood at the koi pond for some time watching the koi swim in and out from under the lily pads. Then I went over to the brick barbeque/smoke oven. Dad used to smoke salmon in the oven, using hickory chips. I opened the oven, and inside it still smelled of hickory and fish. I recalled how, when I was a kid, Dad would peel off a piece of salmon and hand it to me, warm and fresh out of the oven. "Try that," he would say with a big smile. "It doesn't get any better."

Eventually, I went to the living room to see how my mom was doing. An old movie was playing on the TV, a World War II film. The characters on the black-and-white screen were all young men in Navy uniforms. One of the actors was dressed in an officer's uniform, and it reminded me of the pictures I'd seen of my dad during his early Navy days, when Mom and he had started dating. My mom sat staring at the screen—I wasn't sure if she was caught up in the movie, or if she was simply staring through the screen into nothingness.

After a moment, she turned to me and said, "Who called?"

"It was Dr. Wilber," I said.

"Oh?" Mom turned to me with a concerned look on her face. "Is something wrong?"

"No, nothing wrong. He wants to meet with us tomorrow at the hospital. He wants to have a family conference. You, Lori, and me. Two o'clock. I think I like Dr. Wilber."

"He's a good doctor," my mom said.

"He seems to know Dad pretty well. He wants to talk about the next steps."

"Oh?"

"Yeah, after the hospital. He thinks we should bring Dad home. He doesn't like the idea of a nursing home."

"Good." Mom's eyes lit up a little. She took this to be good news. "I don't like that idea, either," she said.

"The thing is," I said, "Dr. Wilber thinks we should bring Dad home because he doesn't think he'd get better in a nursing home. He doesn't think he's going to get better at all."

"Oh," my mom said meekly.

"I think he wants to talk about the feeding tube— whether to leave it in or not. Among other things."

Mom stared at me for a moment. I saw the brief hope of the "homecoming" fade from her eyes. She understood. She slumped into the couch and turned back toward the TV in silence.

"It's just a meeting," I said. "We'll listen to what Wilber has to say. We'll talk about it. Then we'll decide."

Mom said nothing. She just stared at the TV. I sat down next to her on the sofa, and we watched the TV in silence. On the screen, a Navy warship steamed through the large waves of a rough sea filled with white caps.

VII. Conference

The next morning, Mom and I visited Dad at the usual time, 9:00 AM. There were no surprises; condition unchanged. Mom said very little that morning. Previously, she'd made some effort to carry on a conversation, asking how he was doing, telling him some little news from home ("The cat misses you"; "I fed the fish in the koi pond"). This morning, however, she was mostly silent. She simply sat down in her chair and held Dad's hand. I knew she was thinking about the meeting in the afternoon with Dr. Wilber.

I'd contacted my sister; Lori would be there.

I sat down next to Mom. I was thankful there was not another patient in the room. The moment seemed too solemn and private to be shared with strangers. As I watched my father lying there, unable to move or talk, a question floated up in my mind like a stranger stepping out of the fog. It was an uncomfortable question, but a question that had perhaps been kicking around in my unconscious mind: Would it have been better if he had simply died the night he'd had the stroke, at home in his bed? That is, after all, what we all hope for, isn't it? When the time comes, to die peacefully in our sleep.

I tried to imagine Mom's life without Dad. What would she do? She relied so heavily on him. All through their sixty years of marriage, he had been in charge of everything. Mom didn't even know if they had a mortgage on their house. She didn't know cable TV was something you paid for. Dad had handled everything from plumbing problems to balancing her checkbook. How would she cope without him?

At 10:00 AM, the social worker came in. This time I didn't wait for her to ask to talk in private. I stood up and walked out of the room with her, and we went to the nursing station.

"Did you find any nursing homes you might want to consider?" she asked.

"We're probably not going to move my dad to a nursing home," I said.

The social worker looked at me with raised eyebrows.

"We're still thinking about bringing him home," I said. "We're meeting with Dr. Wilber today at 2:00 to talk about it."

"Dr. Wilber?"

"Yes, my dad's regular doctor. He wants to have a family meeting. I talked to him on the phone last night. He's against the nursing home idea."

The eyebrows went up again. "He is?"

"Yes. So, the plan right now is to have the meeting with Wilber. After that, we'll make our decision. I'll let you know."

The social worker fumbled through her jacket pocket and pulled out a business card. "All right," she said handing me her card. "Call me. Take two and give one to Dr. Wilber. I'd like to talk to him."

"Thank you," I said taking the cards. "I will." I stuffed the cards into my pocket and headed back to Dad's room.

*   *   *

Mom and I had lunch at the Fullerton home. Lori arrived at 1:30. We all got in my mom's car and headed for the hospital. We arrived just before 2:00.

As it happened, we ran into Dr. Wilber at the entrance to the main hospital wing. He saw my mom, called out to her, and came over. He was middle-aged, slim and athletic-looking with brown hair just starting to gray at the temples. He was

79

casually dressed in blue jeans, a black polo short, and tennis shoes. The only thing that identified him as a doctor was the stethoscope draped around the back of his neck.

"Hi, Betty," he said solemnly. He reached out his arms and gave her a long hug.

Wilber introduced himself to Lori and me, and we all shook hands. "Good to meet you," he said. "I've heard so much about you both. I feel as though I know you already." He turned back to my mom. "So, what I thought we'd do, Betty, is, first, let's go in and check up on Bill. Is that all right with you?"

"Okay," Mom said. Wilber took her hand, and he escorted her down the hall to my dad's room. "If I'm walking too fast," he said, "let me know. I have a tendency to get ahead of myself if I'm not careful."

We arrived at Dad's room. Wilber pulled three chairs over to the bedside and invited us to sit down. Once we were seated, he turned to my dad. "Hey, Bill," he said putting his hand on Dad's shoulder. "It's Dr. Wilber. How are you doing?"

Dad opened his eyes to the sound of Wilber's voice. You could see, by the slight movement of his head and his eyes, that he was trying to look in the direction of the voice. Wilber leaned over till his face was in front of Dad's eyes. "Here I am. I'm here with Betty, Lori, and Chris. I'd like to check on you while they look on. Is that okay? I hope you don't mind if we talk about you a little bit. I want to explain some of the things while I examine you. Okay?"

Wilber started his exam. While he proceeded, he talked to us and explained what he was doing. It reminded me of medical school days with Wilber playing the part of an attending professor on rounds with a group of medical

80

students. Taking an ophthalmoscope from the mount on the wall, he shined the scope's light into Dad's eyes. "His pupils react well to light," he said to us, "but he doesn't move his eyes to the right. You've probably noticed that."

"Yes," Mom said. "His eyes look funny."

Wilber took a wooden tongue blade out from a drawer next to the bed. "Sorry about this, Bill, but I want to test your gag reflex." He put the blade in Dad's mouth and pressed it against the back of his throat. My dad gagged and coughed a little. "There," Wilber said. "Gag reflex is intact."

Wilber threw the tongue blade in the trash and turned to us. "He still has his gag reflex, and that's a good thing. The problem is, he can't swallow. The stroke has affected the part of the brain that controls swallowing. That means, even with the gag, he's at a high risk to aspirate, to inhale his saliva or anything else in his mouth. It's a guaranteed set up for pneumonia. In fact, he already has pneumonia, and they're giving him antibiotics for that."

Next, Wilber pulled Dad's blankets down and tested the strength in his arms and legs. "He still has a little strength in his left hand, but the right hand is completely flaccid." Wilber lifted Dad's right arm a little off the bed and let it drop. "He's right-handed, as I recall."

"Yes," Mom said.

"Right leg is flaccid, too," Wilber said, "but he's able to move his left leg a little."

Next, Wilber checked Dad's reflexes at the elbows and the knees using the edge of the chest-piece of his stethoscope as a reflex hammer.

"And you thought a stethoscope was just for listening to the heart and lungs," he said glancing at my sister and smiling. "His reflexes are really brisk or what's called 'hyper-reactive.'

81

It's a sign of the stroke and the loss of muscle control." Finally, Wilber checked Dad for the so-called "Babinski sign." Using the non-writing end of an ink pen, he ran the pen over the sole of Dad's right foot. As he did this, Dad's big toe moved upward.

"That's called the Babinski reflex," Wilber said. "You might think it's a good sign to see the toe move up like that. There's some movement there, right? Actually, it's not a good sign. Normally, the toe is supposed to go down. When it goes up, it means there's damage somewhere to the nervous system. In Bill's case, it's another sign of damage to the brain, another sign of his stroke."

Having completed the neurological exam, Wilber proceeded to listen to Dad's heart and lungs with his stethoscope. "He has rhonchi on both sides of the chest," he said. "'Rhonchi' is a fancy word for rattling sounds. It's probably from the pneumonia. Here, Betty, I want you to put your hand on Bill's chest. You can actually feel the rattling. Put your hand here on the right side."

Mom leaned forward in her chair and put the palm of her hand on my dad's chest. "Yes," she said. "I feel it."

"I want you to remember that. We're going to talk more about that. Lori, why don't you feel it, too?"

Lori felt Dad's chest. She nodded her head, indicating that she also felt the rattling.

"Okay, we'll leave you in peace, Bill," Wilber said. He pulled the blankets back up over Dad's chest and smoothed them out. "Betty, Lori, Chris, and I are going to have a talk now. I want to make sure they understand everything that's going on with you. I'll be back later."

Mom stood up and gave Dad a kiss. Wilber took her hand again, and we left the room. We walked down the hall in

82

silence until we reached the family conference room. Wilber opened the door, and we stepped inside. The room contained a large conference table, and I started to sit down in one of the chairs. "Hang on, Chris," Wilber said. "If you don't mind, I prefer to sit in a circle—if that's okay. That conference table is too big and intimidating."

Wilber took four chairs from the table and arranged them in a circle. I sat opposite Wilber; my mom sat on his left, Lori on his right. After a moment of silence, Wilber turned to Mom. "I'm going to direct most of what I have to say to you, Betty, because you're the most important person here. You're the one who has decision-making power when it comes to Bill's care. Not that Chris and Lori aren't important, and I want them to jump in any time if they have a question or a comment or anything to add. But mainly I'm going to focus on you—because you, ultimately, have to make the tough decisions we're going to need to make."

"I want them to help me," Mom said, looking at Lori and me.

"Of course," Wilber said. "That's why Chris and Lori are here—to help. And I'm here to help, too. I'm going to start by just talking a bit about my own history and background, so you can better understand my attitude about what's happening to Bill."

Wilber looked down at the floor for a moment, as though he were drawing upon some inner muse to assist him in what to say. Then he looked up and started:

"When I first started out as a physician, when I was fresh out of residency, I was brim-full with enthusiasm and optimism about being a doctor. I had a head stuffed full of facts, and I thought of myself as being almost invincible. I was going to stamp out illness and disease wherever I saw it. Some of my patients were pretty sick, but that didn't matter—that just increased my eagerness to be a healer. I wanted to save all my patients, even the sickest of them, and make them all better.

"Ah yes, those early days! But…over the years I started to learn I was not all-powerful after all. Nope. Even with all the latest treatments and tools medicine had to offer, there were still some patients who were beyond my reach. There were just some patients I could not make better. It took a while to learn that, and it took even longer to accept it."

Wilber paused to draw again upon his muse. He looked at Lori and me, then back at Mom. He continued:

"I remember a number of years ago, I took care of a physician who'd had a big stroke—just like Bill has had. Just like Bill. He—the physician—and I had been colleagues and friends for a long time. I wanted so badly to help him and to make him whole again. I beat myself up trying to figure out a way to help him. He was much more than a colleague; he was a friend.

"But, there was nothing I could do. Nothing. The stroke had done its damage, and there was no pill or operation or magic potion that could make things better. Like Bill, my physician friend couldn't talk, but I could see in his eyes what he was telling me: 'Don't beat yourself up over it, John. I know. I know there's nothing you can do.'"

Another pause. Wilber went on, looking now down at his hands.

"My own father died six months ago. In a lot of ways, it was the same sort of thing. He'd had a fall and had a bad neck injury. His spinal cord was broken. Same thing—nothing we could do. He died a few days after the injury. There are just some things the best doctors in the world can't fix."

Wilber scooted forward in his chair, looked Mom in the face, and took hold of her hands. "That gurgling in Bill's chest, Betty. That's pneumonia. He got that because he can't swallow. The fluids collect in his mouth, and, when he breathes, he sucks the fluids into his lungs. We can give him antibiotics and cure the pneumonia. But he'll get pneumonia again. And again. Eventually, the antibiotics will stop working because the bacteria will become resistant—the antibiotics will no longer be effective. Do you understand? Does that make sense to you?"

Mom looked at Lori and me. She looked back at Wilber. "I think so," she said.

"I know Bill doesn't want to be in a nursing home. I know that because he said that to me, literally, in my office: 'Dr. Wilber, I don't ever want to be in a nursing home. Don't ever let anyone do that to me.' And I also know it because of the other conversations we had. I'm thinking specifically about a conversation we had about Bill's ranch.

"You know, he sort of measured his health by how much he could do at the ranch. Seriously, he did. He worried about the arthritis in his knees and how it was limiting his activities. But, as long as he could take care of his cattle—toss them some hay, herd them into the barn in the winter—then life was worth living.

"However—and, again, he told me this—he said: 'If I ever get to the point where I can't take care of my cows, then life is no longer worth living.' He was being metaphorical about the cows, of course. It's not that he was saying taking care of cows was the only important thing in his life. But this was his way of gauging the minimal level of health he considered necessary to...to keep on living. It was a sort of code he used."

Wilber gave Mom's hands another squeeze. "Does that sound like Bill?" he asked.

"Yes," she said softly.

Wilber looked at Lori.

"Yes," Lori said.

"Chris?" Wilber said. "Sounds like your dad?"

I nodded my head.

"I'll tell you one other conversation Bill and I had. It's a little delicate, but it's relevant to what we're talking about right now. Bill said to me, if he ever got so sick that he couldn't live the active life he wanted to live, then he wanted me to give him a pill or a shot…something that would put him asleep—forever."

Wilber paused to let this sink in. Then he went on.

"That's what he wanted. A pill. He called it 'death with dignity.' Of course, I told him I couldn't do that. It's not legal, not in the state of California, anyway. But I did make him a promise. While I couldn't give him that pill or that shot he wanted, I promised I would never act to prolong his suffering either. If he ever became ill, and if I saw there was no hope that he'd get better, then I promised I would not give him any medications or treatments that I knew he didn't want. I know that's hard for you to hear, Betty, but that's how he felt. He felt strongly about that. That's the conversation we had."

My mom nodded her head, indicating she understood. Frankly, I was surprised by how well she was holding up so far.

"Bill can't talk for himself now," Wilber said. "That's why I feel a moral obligation to speak on his behalf. I know you're thinking about putting him in a nursing home, but I believe that is not what Bill would want. Not in a million years. I'll be very honest with you, Betty: Bill is not going to be taking care of those cows at his ranch ever again. Never. I know that's hard, but it's the truth. And I'll tell you what else. I do not believe Bill would want to be kept alive artificially in the state he's in now. I know that because I know Bill. What I'm saying, Betty…what I'm saying is…I believe what Bill really wants is to come home and let go."

Mom's bottom lip began to tremble. Of course, she understood what Wilber meant by "let go."

"I'm speaking for Bill, now," Wilber said. "I believe he wants to be in his own home, surrounded by his own family. He doesn't want to waste away and eventually die in some nursing home, in some unfamiliar room shared with another person, surrounded by strangers. You know what else I think, Betty? I don't think he wants all the IVs and that tube in his nose. He doesn't want any of that. Not any more."

Another pause. Wilber was still holding Mom's hands.

"My recommendation," Wilber said softly, "is we bring Bill home and put him under the care of a team called hospice. They would come to your home and help care for him—and help you. There would be a nurse, attendants, a clergyman if you want. The hospice people are experts at what's called 'comfort care.' They would give Bill all the medicines he needed to be comfortable. But no treatments to keep him alive artificially. And—just so you understand exactly what I'm saying—over the course of a few days at home, without food and water, Bill would start to drift in and out of consciousness. The periods of unconsciousness would get longer and longer. If there were ever any signs of pain, he would be given pain medication. He would probably hang on for maybe a week, maybe a bit longer. Then he would peacefully pass away. In his own home, surrounded by his family. That, in my opinion, is what Bill wants."

Mom looked at Dr. Wilber but said nothing. There were

87

tears in her eyes. Wilber got up and pulled a tissue from a Kleenex box on the conference table, and he handed it to my mom.

After a long period of silence, Wilber turned to Lori and me. "The choice is up to the three of you. We'll do whatever you want. I know that, financially, Bill is in pretty good shape, and we could find him a nursing home where he would get good care. I'll help you out with that if that's the choice you make. I just felt I had to stand in and give a pitch for what I believe are your dad's wishes. Do you, Chris, or you, Lori, think I'm getting it wrong?"

"He never talked us," I said, "not to me, anyway, about it. But I think what you're saying sounds right. I found a file in his desk at home. It's called 'Hemlock.' It has information about exactly what you're talking about: hospice care, dying at home. Also, he sometimes talked about how he never wanted to die like his mom…."

"I know about that," Wilber said. "Your dad told me."

I had a question. "Dr. Alexander told us," I said, "that although my dad can't express himself, he still understands. Is it possible to communicate with him some way other than verbally? You know, like have him squeeze your hand, once for 'yes' twice for 'no.' Something like that."

"Actually, I tried that," Wilber said. "He can't do it. Nice thought, though. It's not just his verbal expression that got cut off by the stroke. It's all communication output; it's called a global expressive aphasia. It's like typing into a computer with a blank screen. You can type in the input, but you can't see the output. Unfortunately, your dad just can't tell us what he wants. He can't help us out. The best we can do is base our decisions on what we know about your dad and on what he's told us in the past."

88

Wilber turned to my sister. "Any thoughts, Lori? You've been pretty quiet."

Lori shifted in her chair. "It's just…it's just hard—bring him home and do nothing. I mean—just watch him—what?—starve?"

"I know, it's hard," Wilber said, "but I didn't say do nothing. We'd be doing everything possible to make him comfortable. That would include giving him sedating medication and pain medication like morphine. And, no, he would not starve. Most likely his pneumonia would get worse, because he would continue to aspirate germs into his lungs. But is pneumonia necessarily a bad thing? You know, in the old days, they used to call pneumonia 'the old man's friend.' Seriously. Pneumonia was seen as a swift and gentle end to life. The lungs fill up with fluid, less and less oxygen to the brain, loss of consciousness and, before long…. It's a relatively peaceful way to go."

Lori said nothing.

"I don't expect you to make a decision right now," Wilber said. "Go home, talk about it, the three of you. It's a very big decision, obviously—don't let anyone rush you. We could even have Bill transferred to a nursing home temporarily if you want. There's no law that says Bill couldn't be in a nursing for a week or two while you make up your mind."

With that, Wilber stood up. He bent down and put his hands on my mom's shoulders. "So, Betty," he said, "I'm going to go write a note in Bill's chart now. I've said my piece. You can stay here as long as you like and talk. Call me anytime, day or night, with questions. If you want to meet and sit down and talk again, just let me know."

He leaned down and hugged her. My mom hugged him back in silence. Straightening up, Wilber looked at my sister

89

and me. "Nice meeting you, Chris, Lori." He shook our hands. "Same goes with you: call anytime. If you reach a decision or if you have any questions, call."

With that, Wilber headed toward the door.

I knew he'd told us the truth. He'd done his best to advocate for what he thought were my father's wishes, and he'd done so in a kind, unhurried, and compassionate way. I was impressed. What a contrast to the icy Dr. Alexander and the freeze-dried ICU nurse. He was exactly the sort of doctor we needed at that moment. He knew my father, and he knew him well. He knew my mother, too, and I could tell she trusted him.

"Dr. Wilber," I called out as he started to out the door.

Wilber stopped and turned back.

"Thanks," I said, giving him a nod. "Just...thanks."

VIII. Decision

After the family meeting with Dr. Wilber, Mom, Lori, and I went back to the house in Fullerton. We made coffee and tea, and we went to the living room. We sat together on the sofa, and we talked. We were about to make one of the most difficult decisions any of us would ever have to make.

We first tackled the easy part, the nursing home question: Yes or no? The vote was quick and unanimous. No nursing home. There was no doubt in anyone's mind: my dad would never want to live out his final days in a nursing home. Never. Despite the recommendation and warnings voiced by the social worker, we all agreed: Dad was coming home.

That was easy. Now came the hard part—the nearly impossible part. What would be the plan for him once we got him home?

I knew Dr. Wilber had spoken honestly for my dad, especially the part about his saying life wouldn't be worth living if he became severely disabled. Something about that rang true. An active life had always been of supreme importance to Dad. When I was growing up, he used to come into my room and drag me out of bed if I slept past 8:00 in the morning. "Get up! You're wasting good daylight!"

I knew that, to my father, a life of inactivity would be intolerable. I pictured him now in his hospital bed, paralyzed, the NG tube in his nose. He could not communicate his wishes to us, but in my gut I knew he would not want to live a life confined to a bed, fed by a tube, completely dependent on others to turn him, feed him, bathe him. If he were able to talk, I knew what he would say to us. He would tell us he did not want to slowly die a prisoner in his own bed, a captive trapped inside his own broken body. *If I ever get to the point where I can't take care of my cows, then life is no longer worth living.*

"I'm going to side with Dr. Wilber," I said to my mom and my sister. "Bring him home on hospice. I think that's what he would want."

After a moment of silence, my sister said, "What about the feeding tube?"

"I vote no," I said. "All it would do is…prolong things."

"Yeah, but—if he's going to get pneumonia anyway," Lori said, "at least we can feed him."

"But is that what *he* would want?" I said. "That's the most important question. We should do what he would want us to do."

"We don't know what he wants," my sister said. "He can't talk."

"I think we do know," I said. "You heard what Wilber said. They talked about this—if he got the way he is now. Plus…I should show you something. Remember that Hemlock file I talked about?"

"Yeah?" Lori said.

"I want you to look at it."

I went to Dad's study, got the file, and brought it back into the living room.

"It's about end-of-life stuff," I said. I handed the file to Mom. "There are articles about hospice and exactly the sort of thing Wilber was talking about."

My mom opened the file. The first thing she saw was the *Time* magazine with the dying man on the cover.

"I don't like this," she said. "Here. I don't want it." She handed the file back to me. I handed it over to my sister.

Lori went through the file. The picture on the cover of *Time* had shaken up Mom, and she wiped her eyes with a

Kleenex. After a couple of minutes, my sister closed the file folder and put it down on the coffee table.

"Okay," she said.

"Did Dad ever talk about it with you?"

"No," Lori said.

I looked at my mom. "Mom?"

"No," she replied.

"Remember how he said he didn't want to die like his mother?" I asked.

"Yes," my mom said. "I remember."

I picked up the Hemlock file and held it up. "*This* is him talking to us. I think this is what he wants. He knew we would find this. It's in the main file drawer of his desk. Of course we're going to look there."

My sister and my mom remained silent.

"If these are his wishes," I said, "then that's what we should go by." I asked Mom: "Would he want a feeding tube? Confined to bed, unable to walk or move? You know Dad. He thinks you're a slouch if you aren't out of bed doing something productive by sunrise. He used to make fun of me when I went jogging. 'Why waste your time jogging? Go out and dig a ditch. You get just as much exercise, and you accomplish something.'"

My mom did not respond.

"We have to decide something," I said. "We have to tell the hospital people what we want to do. They're going to discharge him pretty soon."

"No nursing home," Mom said.

"Yes, we all agree on that," I said. "But what about the feeding tube?" I looked at my mom. I looked at my sister. The feeding tube had become the crux of the hard decision we were trying to make, a metaphor for life versus death.

"I can't say take it out," Mom said. "It's too hard."

"I know it's hard," I said softly.

"It's the same as saying, 'Kill him. Kill him!'" my mom blurted out. Her head fell back, and she closed her eyes. "I don't want to talk about it anymore."

I put my arm around her. There was a long period of silence.

"You decide," she finally said. "I can't. I *can't!*"

"How about this?" I said after a moment. "It's a compromise. Bring him home, and bring him home on hospice. Comfort care, right? But, we leave the feeding tube in. We decide after he gets home if we want to use it. Maybe we'll go a day or two without the feeds. But say he starts to improve. Bringing him home on hospice doesn't mean we *can't* ever feed him. If he starts to improve, the hospice nurse can bring feeding supplies and set up a pump—they do that all the time—*if we want it.* We'll leave that as an option. But, for now, we get Dad home, get him out of the hospital and into his own bed in his own house. How does that sound?"

"Yes," my mom immediately said. "I want to bring him home."

"Lori?" I said. "Bring him home. Leave the tube in. But decide after a day or two if we want to use it."

"All right." There was some reluctance in her tone. Nevertheless, she repeated: "All right. Yeah."

"But, just so we have it clear," I said, "the initial plan is no feeds. I'll need to let the hospice people know. We bring him home, and we reserve the right to use the tube if we decide to later."

"Yes," my mother said. "I like that."

I could see that her main focus was on bringing Dad home. In addition, she liked the idea of leaving the tube in. It was a bit of a copout: we had, essentially, decided not to decide. *Leave the tube in but don't use it.* But I understood the equivocation. There *was* something terribly difficult about pulling the tube. The *feeding* tube. To purposely hold back on something as basic as food and water—to imagine my father suffering the pangs of hunger and thirst—it was such a basic instinct to want to provide nutrition to a loved one.

Moreover, taking out the tube made things so final. It was a complete capitulation (even though, in reality, the tube could always be replaced), and no one was quite ready for that. Even *I* felt a certain comfort in leaving the tube in. By leaving it in, we were still clinging to a slim reed of optimism. Maybe, despite all expectations, Dad would improve. And if he did, the tube would be there, ready for use, ready to sustain his life. It was a symbol of hope.

Without saying anything more, I left my mom and my sister in the living room and went to Dad's study. There in private, I called Dr. Wilber and let him know our decision.

IX. Hospice

The next day, we arrived at the hospital at the usual time, 9:00 AM. Dad was lying on his side, the sheets pulled up to his nose, his eyes peeking out, looking to the left and up at the ceiling. Condition unchanged. The pump on the feeding tube was running; the milky, light-brown solution dripped slowly from the bottle into the NG tube. Antibiotic fluid dripped from a plastic bag hanging from an IV pole.

Mom sat down at the side of the bed and took hold of his hand. "Hi Bill," she said pulling the sheet down off his face. "Oh, you've gotten a shave! Look how *good* you look."

Mom was right: in between when we'd left the hospital yesterday afternoon and now, someone had shaved Dad. It was the first shave he'd had since being admitted to St Mark's, and the removal of the gray stubble from his face significantly improved his appearance. His hair looked clean and neatly combed as well.

Just then, the social worker arrived. "I understand there's going to be a homecoming," she said cheerfully at the doorway.

"Yes," I said, standing up. She and I left the room and went to the nursing station, just as we'd done on the previous two mornings.

"You want to take him home, then," the social worker said. "On hospice."

"Yes, we do. We had a long talk with Dr. Wilber yesterday, and he felt that was the best thing. My mom, my sister, and I talked it over, and we all agree. Home on hospice. The one thing is we want to leave the NG tube in for now. We're not planning on using it, but if we change our mind…."

"That's perfectly fine. Sure. All that can be worked out with hospice."

I was surprised at how agreeable the social worker was. I'd thought she might persist in trying to talk us into a nursing home. I also thought she might express bewilderment over the idea of leaving the NG tube in. However, there was no hesitation or pushback. The social worker seemed perfectly comfortable with "the plan."

"So, the next step," she said, "is choosing a hospice provider. There are several here in Orange County."

She took a piece of paper from her canvas shoulder bag and handed it to me. It was a list of hospice providers providing services in Fullerton, including contact information.

"Do you have a recommendation?" I asked, scanning the list.

"We're not allowed to make recommendations," the social worker said. "However, I think I'm allowed to say Odyssey is the most popular. By far."

Odyssey Health Care was the third company on the list. They had an office in the area. There was a phone number and a website.

"Any complaints or problems you know of?" I asked.

"Nope."

"We'll go with them, then," I said. It was probably irresponsible of me to make a snap decision like that. I should have taken the list home, checked the websites, made some phone calls, looked into testimonials. However, although the social worker was not supposed to recommend any particular provider, it seemed pretty clear Odyssey was her first choice.

"All right," the social worker said. "I'll contact them and let them know of your interest and the situation. What'll happen is they'll contact you and set up an interview. They usually like to come out and talk to you at your house. It gives them a chance to look over the home situation and the environment they'll be working in."

"Sounds good," I said.

"Should I have them call you or your mom?"

"Me."

The social worker seemed so pleasant and cheerful now that we had a definitive discharge plan. I knew that one of her chief job tasks was to effect a smooth release from the hospital when patients were ready to leave. Our decision to bring Dad home had put us on the path to task completion.

I gave her my contact information and went back to Dad's room.

"She's the social worker, remember?" I said to Mom. "I told her we want to bring him home. She's going to arrange it."

"Good," Mom said.

I leaned forward and spoke loudly to Dad. "We're going to bring you home, Dad. Probably tomorrow. Home to Fullerton. What do you think about that?"

It might have been my imagination, but something brightened in the look on his face, something in the expression in his eyes. I think he was smiling.

*   *   *

Early that afternoon, back at the Fullerton house, Odyssey Health Care called. I spoke to a man named Mike who identified himself as the owner of the local Odyssey branch. He asked if he could come out to the house later in the day in order to talk to us about the program. We set up an appointment. Mike arrived punctually, ringing the doorbell at

4:00. He was a short, muscular man with brown hair and a small moustache. He wore a dark blue polo shirt and carried a clipboard with medical forms. Introductions were made, and Mike, my mother, and I sat down in the living room.

Mike began by giving us some information about himself. He had been a respiratory therapist for over fifteen years before starting the Orange County branch of Odyssey. He'd been involved in hospice care for over seven years now and said all the members of his staff were experienced hospice caregivers.

Next, he gave a careful and clear definition of hospice. "Hospice," he said, "is compassionate, supportive care for patients with a terminal diagnosis. The focus is on dignity and comfort, including pain management. Hospice care, however, is not curative care. If you're looking for a cure, we're not for you." Mike looked at Mom and then at me.

"We understand," I said.

"All hospice patients are assigned a team that includes a nurse, a physician, home health aides, and a social worker. A chaplain is also available. We provide any and all equipment that might be needed. Now, I understand Mr. Stookey has had a stroke. He's unable to walk or move much. He can't swallow. Non-verbal."

"That's correct," I said.

"Obviously he'll need a hospital bed with an air mattress, oxygen, a suction machine. Medicare covers all our services, by the way, including equipment. Most patients and their families are surprised to hear that. Everything we do is covered. There's no cost to you. Zero."

I *was* surprised to hear this. Although money wasn't a huge issue for us, it was nice to know Medicare would pick up the tab. I suspected there was a time limit on how long

Medicare would cover the hospice care. Time, however, would probably not be an issue.

Not if we didn't use the feeding tube.

"I'm going to assign Marcia as your nurse," Mike said. "Great nurse, fantastic. One of our best. I'll have her call you later this evening and go over the plan. My understanding is you're wanting to bring Mr. Stookey home tomorrow."

"Um, we hadn't set a day yet," I said. "But, yeah, tomorrow is good."

"Could I see the room you'll be putting him in?" Mike asked.

"Sure." My mom and I had decided on the bedroom. At first I'd thought the best room might be my dad's study—that was the room where he previously had spent most of his waking hours. His TV and stereo were in the study, and there was a nice view of the backyard. However, it would be a tight squeeze getting a hospital bed into the study, and there wouldn't be much room to maneuver. Plus, the bedroom was in a quieter, more private part of the house. It seemed a more logical choice.

I showed Mike the bedroom. "Yes, this is fine," he said. He told us the delivery crew would move the queen bed that was there now to make room for the hospital bed. "Do you know where you'll want to store the queen?"

"In the garage," I said.

"Perfect. Just let the delivery crew know."

We went back to the living room. The final item of business was paperwork. There were triplicate forms giving Odyssey permission to enter our home and provide all manner of hospice care for William Stookey. There was authorization for the equipment: the bed, air mattress, air mattress pump, oxygen tank, suction pump, suction catheters, a wheelchair (this last item was something I didn't think we'd be needing, but I didn't quibble). Mike briefly explained each form, and my mom signed the papers.

"We'll have the equipment delivered tomorrow morning," Mike said. "Don't worry, we'll coordinate everything with the hospital. We'll have all the equipment in and the room set up before William comes home, probably sometime in the early afternoon."

Mike gave us a notebook containing copies of the paperwork and contact numbers. Hospice personnel would be available to take our calls twenty-four hours a day. He also gave us a spiral-bound booklet, "The Handbook of Hospice," describing everything from hospice philosophy to home safety. In addition, he gave us a smaller booklet called, "Gone From My Sight." As I would later discover, this booklet described the process of dying and what to expect as a loved one approached death. I gathered up all the material, placed it in a stack on the living room table, and escorted Mike to the door.

"Someone from Odyssey will update you on the exact time to expect your dad home tomorrow," Mike said. "Marcia will bring by all the medications you'll need—the medicines to give your dad to keep him comfortable."

"Thanks," I said. "You've been very thorough."

"We try to cover all the bases. Anyway, Marcia will be calling you later on. Bye, Chris."

I said goodbye and went back into the house. Walking into the living room, I saw my mom had turned on the television. Turner Classic Movies. It seemed these old movies gave her some comfort. Or perhaps they just diverted her mind from thinking about what was too hard for her to think about. I was going to go over and sit next to her, but there was something about her posture and the look on her face—she didn't look up at me when I came back into the room—that suggested she wanted to be alone.

I decided to go the bedroom and to get things ready for Dad's arrival.

*   *   *

As promised, Marcia called early in the evening. By her voice, she sounded to be fairly young—perhaps in her mid-thirties. She asked for me by name, and it was quickly apparent she knew all the important details about my dad. She said she'd already been in touch with the nurses at St. Mark's. They had told her my dad's condition was "very endstage," as she put it, and they agreed with our decision to bring my dad home on hospice.

She told me she would meet us at the house shortly after my dad arrived home tomorrow at around 1:00 PM. She would bring, among other things, a "comfort kit." "It contains morphine and Ativan along with other comfort drugs," she said. "Morphine for pain, Ativan as a sedative. The two work very well together."

We also talked about the NG tube.

"My mom can't bring herself to have it removed," I said. "We'd like to leave it in…just in case we change our mind."

"No problem. That's actually quite common," Marcia said. "Families do that all the time. The feeding tube is like a lifeline, and emotionally it's hard to say 'throw away the lifeline.'"

I found it somehow reassuring that other families were similarly ambivalent about removing the feeding tube, and that Marcia understood this. I appreciated that she didn't try to talk us into taking it out, she didn't point out that we were acting irrationally, she didn't pass judgment about our indecisiveness. I liked her already.

*   *   *

That evening, Mom and I went to visit Dad for the last time in the hospital. Another patient now occupied the other bed in the room, and there were several people gathered around the newcomer's bed talking, eating, and laughing. They were a noisy group.

I closed the curtain between the two beds, and Mom and I sat down with Dad. He seemed a little agitated, moving his leg and blinking his eyes. I'm sure it was due to the noise and the other people in the room. Every now and then one of the visitors on the other side of the curtain would let out a loud laugh, and Dad would turn his head in the direction of the noise. The expressive side of his face appeared vaguely distressed. I don't know what the diagnosis was for the man in the next bed, but whatever it was, he didn't seem terribly sick. His voice was vigorous, cheerful, and as loud as the others. Each time he laughed or talked, it emphasized the contrast between his more verbal and hearty condition and my Dad's condition. Peevishly, I thought the hospital admissions people should be more careful in how they went about choosing roommates.

We stayed with Dad for an hour. It was a subdued visit. I told him again of the plan to bring him home tomorrow. I'm not sure if he understood me or not; he seemed more attentive to the noises next door. My mom said almost nothing the entire time. She simply sat at the side of the bed holding his hand. At times she stared lovingly into his face; at times she stared blankly off into space. At one point I noted tears in her eyes. Of course, I knew she was thinking about the homecoming tomorrow. The homecoming. It should have been a joyous occasion—any homecoming should be. This one, however, would be different.

The other people let out a cheer. They were watching a basketball game on the TV. The team they were rooting for must have just scored a crucial point. Once again, Dad turned his head in the direction of the noise.

I leaned forward and put my hand on my dad's chest. "Don't worry," I said in a voice loud enough for the people next door to hear. "Tomorrow you'll be back in your own bed. Tomorrow you'll be back home."

X. Homecoming

They came with the equipment mid-morning, two burly men in a van. They brought in the hospital bed and set it up in the bedroom. They put an air mattress on the bed and filled it using a compressor pump; the mattress rubber creaked and popped as it inflated. Next came the large, green oxygen tank that the men set up next to the bed. They attached a line of plastic tubing to the tank and draped the pronged end of the line over the head of the bed, ready for use. They brought in a suction machine, put it on a table next to the bed, and turned it on to test the suction. The pump made a noise like a muffled sewing machine.

The men brought in a variety of other supplies: diapers, towels, body wipes, bed sheets, gloves, basins, lotions, bed chucks, alcohol swipes, sponge lollipops (little blue sponge cubes on a stick for moistening the mouth). I was impressed. They—hospice, that is—had thought of everything. At the same time, the sight of all this medical equipment gave me a sick feeling in my stomach. Suction machine, oxygen tank, diapers, bed chucks—these were not the things of a happy homecoming.

Before leaving, the men made the bed. They put on new, white sheets with perfect hospital corners and the sheets precisely turned down, ready for Dad's arrival. Mom and I supplied the blankets and pillowcases; we topped the bed with Dad's favorite green comforter.

Before leaving, the two men showed me how to use the bed controls. There was a button to raise the head and another button to lift the legs up and down. The men were polite, friendly, and appropriately somber—just the right demeanor

105

for the occasion. It's funny how, given the situation, you appreciate little things like that.

After the men left, we added some final touches to the room. We put a bouquet of flowers in a vase on the dresser across from the bed, fall colors: roses, daisies, and mini-carnations; red, yellow, and orange. We set up a small fan on the bedside table. I turned the nightstand radio on to Dad's favorite station, 91.5 FM, the twenty-four-hour classical music station. I opened the window to the backyard to let in some fresh air. The sound of the koi pond waterfall came in through the window.

With everything set up and ready to go, Mom and I went into the living room and waited. It was 12:30. The plan was for Dad to come home by ambulance at one o'clock. I sipped a cup of black coffee and looked out the window. My mom sat and stared down at the floor, mostly. I'd made her a cup of tea, but she hadn't touched it. She wasn't doing well. Although she wanted Dad to come home, she knew what lay ahead. Every time a car passed by on the street, she looked up with a start. I finished my coffee and asked Mom if she wanted a warm-up on her tea. "No thanks," she said, looking down at her cup. It was still full to the brim.

At exactly one o'clock, they pulled up into the driveway in a white-and-blue ambulance. There was the driver and another medic in the back of the rig with Dad. Mom looked surprised and troubled—I don't think she'd understood they would bring him home by ambulance. I stood on the porch and watched as the medics carefully rolled Dad out on a stretcher. He was lying on his back, covered by a tan blanket with belt straps across his chest and thighs. They wheeled him to the porch, lifted him up the two steps, and rolled him in through the front door.

For the first time in six days, Dad was back in his own home. I'm convinced I saw a spark of emotion light up on the good side of his face: the corner of his mouth turned up slightly, and there was a twinkle in his eyes. He was smiling. Even the paramedics saw it, and they smiled back at him. Mom, looking suddenly happy for the first time since my dad's stroke, saw it, too.

"Are you happy to be home?" she said, kissing him on the cheek. "You are, aren't you?"

I led the paramedics into the bedroom, and they parked Dad next to the bed. They adjusted the height of the gurney so it was level with the bed and carefully transferred him from the stretcher to the bed. They put one pillow under his knees and another under his head. They'd been giving him oxygen for the ambulance ride, and now they took away their oxygen tubing and replaced it with the new tubing that was draped over the head of the bed. They hooked Dad's Foley catheter bag onto the side of the bed; I noticed it was a quarter-full with urine. One of the medics turned on the oxygen flow from the green tank.

The other medic took a clipboard from the stretcher, made an "X" on one of the papers, and handed the clipboard to me. "If you'll just sign here. It's so we can bill his insurance for the ride from the hospital." I signed the paper, and the medic tore off a copy for me. "All set, then," he said. "The hospital called the hospice nurse and let her know we were leaving. She said she'd be here in about an hour."

"All right, Mr. Stookey," the other medic said to Dad. He squeezed his shoulder. "You take care, then, okay?"

Dad was moving his head slightly from side to side, looking around the bedroom. His bedroom. It was as though he wanted to take in as much of it as he could. The "smile" on his face was still there. I walked the medics to the front door and thanked them. Shutting the door, I started back for the bedroom.

Halfway down the hallway, however, I stopped. I realized that something didn't feel right. Now that the paramedics had left, a stillness weighed down on the walls of the house. There was an odd—almost an eerie—quiet in the air. After a moment, I understood what was wrong. My dad had always been the central force of energy in the family, and now that he was back home, I'd expected the power of that force to re-ignite just by his physical presence. But it was not to be. Even though my dad was physically home, his presence did not fill up the house the way it had for over fifty years. There was neither the sound of his voice, nor the sound of his footsteps, nor even the simple force of his being. There was only the stillness.

I made my way back into the bedroom, where Mom and I fussed over Dad for half an hour. My mom combed his hair and fluffed his pillows. I adjusted the volume on the radio and tested the suction machine, suctioning out his mouth secretions. I fiddled with the bed controls, moving his head up and down until I had him positioned just right. I remember that Vivaldi's *Four Seasons* was playing on the radio.

Despite the "stillness," it was good to have my dad home again. I took hold of his hand and smiled at him. "It's good to have you back," I said. "Good to have you back."

*   *   *

At 2:15, the doorbell rang. It was Marcia. I let her in, and we shook hands. As I'd guessed from our phone conversation, she was in her mid-thirties. She had blonde, shoulder-length hair, and she looked neat and professional in her white coat and black-rimmed glasses. She was carrying a dark grey satchel that hung from a strap over her shoulder.

I thought we would go straight in and check on Dad. Instead, Marcia asked if she could sit down and talk with Mom and me first.

We sat down in the living room and talked for ten minutes. Marcia asked about how we were doing emotionally. She emphasized that her job was to make sure Dad was made as comfortable as possible, but she would also do everything she could to help all of us through this difficult period.

"I spoke with the nurses at the hospital," she said. "They said Bill's stroke is quite severe. I know how hard this is for you." She opened her satchel and took out a white box about the size of a shoebox. "This," she said, "is a 'comfort kit.' It contains the medicines we'll need to keep Bill comfortable. Chris, I understand you're a physician."

"Yes," I said.

"That's lucky. A lot of times, family members find all this—especially the medications—a bit overwhelming." Marcia opened the box and took out two small bottles. "These are your two most important medicines. Morphine, which of course is for pain; Ativan for agitation and anxiety."

Marcia explained that the medicines came in liquid form and were to be given via a dropper inserted under the tongue. Dad would not have to swallow the medicine; the membranes of his mouth would absorb it. Marcia took a notebook out and gave us a chart showing how much medicine to give and how often.

"The dose can be adjusted according to how much pain or agitation Bill seems to be having. Most people err on the side of giving too little. They're afraid they'll give an overdose.

In my ten years of nursing, I've never seen that happen. In other words, don't be afraid to give the higher dose if needed."

There were other items in the kit, and Marcia went over them all. There was a suppository for nausea, another for fever, another for constipation. There was a dropper bottle containing atropine.

"Give him a couple drops of the atropine every two hours, and it'll dry up his mouth secretions," she said. "He won't choke as much. If his mouth and lips get too dry, moisten them with a sponge lollipop dipped in water."

Marcia put everything back in the kit and handed the box to me. She closed her satchel and folded her hands in her lap. "So. What do you say we go in and meet Bill?"

I led the way into the bedroom. Looking back, I noticed the lost look on my mom's face as she followed behind us. Dad was awake, his eyes open. Marcia went straight to the head of the bed, took his hand, and introduced herself.

"Hi, Bill, I'm Marcia. I'm the nurse from Odyssey Healthcare, and I'm going to help Betty and Chris take care of you." She positioned herself so Dad could see her with his leftward-gazing eyes. "How are you doing?" she asked, leaning down and speaking loudly. "Are you comfortable?"

"He's not able to talk at all," I said.

"I know, they told me at St. Mark's," Marcia said. She looked at Mom and me. "But I think he understands."

"That's what the neurologist told us," I said.

Marcia turned back to Dad. "I'll bet you're happy to be home, eh Bill?"

She proceeded to do a brief neurological exam, checking the strength of Dad's arms and legs and testing his reflexes. "He has a little strength on his left side," she said as she proceeded through the exam, "but it's not enough to allow him to turn from side to side in bed. He's going to be at a risk for pressure sores. Chris, can you help me roll him, so I can check the condition of his skin in back?"

Using the bed controls, I lowered my dad's head. Then we rolled him up on his side. He was still wearing a hospital gown, and Marcia opened the gown in back and pulled down his diapers.

"His skin is in pretty good condition," she said. "Sometimes that's not the case when they come home from the hospital." We rolled Dad back over on his back. "Avoiding pressure sores is going to be one of our biggest jobs," Marcia said. "Bill needs to be turned every two hours. Day and night. I know that's not going to be easy. The air mattress will help, but there's still a lot of weight on his lower back and buttock area. Also on his heels. Those are the danger points."

Next, Marcia turned her attention to Dad's mouth secretions. She took a penlight out of her satchel and looked inside his mouth. "Oh, boy. Lots of saliva," she said. She turned on the suction machine and placed the plastic suction catheter in his mouth. "You don't want to put the catheter too far in," she said over the loud sound of the suctioning. "Most of the secretions will pool between his cheeks and his teeth. Chris, do you mind giving me those atropine drops?"

Marcia spent another half hour with Dad, propping him up on pillows, adjusting his bed, taking his blood pressure and temperature, and recording the amount of urine in his Foley bag. All the while, she talked to my dad, explaining what she was doing. When she was finished, she put away her things in her satchel.

"Well—it was very good to meet you, Bill," she said. "Everything here looks great." She gave him a hug, and, then, with her hands still on his shoulders, she said, "You look very comfortable, and we're going to keep you that way. Okay? I'll be back tomorrow, same time. All right? See you then!"

We went back to the living room and sat down. I asked Marcia if she wanted some coffee or tea. She declined. She took a couple minutes to write some things down in a notebook, then she turned to my mom and said: "Betty? You've been very quiet. I know all this is pretty overwhelming. Are you okay?"

"Oh…as good as I can be," Mom said, looking down at her hands.

"It's hard to see Bill this way, isn't it? How long have you been married?"

"Fifty-two years," Mom said.

"Wow. I'll bet at least you're happy he's home. And, I'll bet Bill's happy to be home, too."

"Yes, he is," Mom said. "I can tell."

"He's comfortable, Betty." Marcia took my mom's hands in hers. "He's comfortable, and we're going to keep him that way. Okay?"

Mom did not reply.

"Would you like to have our chaplain visit?" Marcia asked. "We have a non-denominational chaplain. He's very good."

"I'll think about it," Mom said. "Not right now."

"There's also our social worker," Marcia added. "She can help you work through the difficult emotions everyone feels at a time like this. That's what she's there for."

"Thank you," Mom said. "But I don't want anyone right now."

"Okay, sure," Marcia said. She turned back toward me. "You've got my phone number, Chris. I'm available twenty-four hours a day. Normally, I don't let my calls roll over to the

112

Odyssey hot line—I take them directly. So, call me anytime with questions, concerns, changes in Bill's condition. Anything. I don't care if it's 3:00 in the morning."

Marcia stood up and put her satchel strap over her shoulder. "I'll be back tomorrow." She leaned down and gave Mom a hug. "'Bye, Betty."

I walked Marcia to the door. I liked her. She was professional but also very warm—and obviously quite experienced. I felt lucky we'd gotten her as our nurse. "Thanks," I said at the door. "See you tomorrow, then."

"Look after your mom," Marcia said. "I'm a little worried about her. She seems a little withdrawn and kind of unsure about what's happening."

"Yeah," I said. "I know."

"It might not be a bad idea to have our social worker pay her a visit."

"I'll talk to her about it," I said. "I'll let you know."

"Okay. See you tomorrow, Chris." Marcia started down the steps.

"Thanks again," I said. "See you tomorrow."

XI. Vigil

After Marcia left, I went into the bedroom and sat with Dad. I moved the comfortable blue armchair over to the side of the bed and settled into it with "The Handbook of Hospice." My dad had fallen asleep, no doubt worn out after his five-and-a-half-day ordeal in the hospital. He probably hadn't slept much in the hospital, first under the bright lights of the ICU and later in the room shared with the noisy family.

I read through the handbook, going through the sections on skin care, pain control, and comfort measures. Putting down the book, I reviewed the directions Marcia had written out for the administration of the morphine:

A quarter dropper full (5 milligrams) every 2 hours as needed for mild pain;

A half dropper full (10 milligrams) every 2 hours as needed for moderate pain;

A full dropper full (20 milligrams) every 2 hours as needed for severe pain.

I was fully ready to give the morphine at the first indication my father was having any pain.

At 5:00, I turned him. I was able to do it on my own. He was still asleep, and I gently shook his shoulder to wake him. "Dad," I said. "Dad." He opened his eyes and looked around the best he could in the direction of my voice. "Sorry to wake you up. I have to turn you over. We need to do it every two hours." I was going to say "so you don't get bedsores," but I remembered his mother's death and his fear of bedsores. I decided not to mention the word.

114

I lowered the head of the bed and removed the pillows propping him up on his left side. Going around to the other side of the bed, I pushed him up on his opposite side and stuffed the pillows under his upper and lower back. It was like moving dead weight, and my dad was so limp he tended to slide off the pillows. I pushed him up with the heel of one hand and stuffed the pillows deep under him with the other. I could see how it would be much easier to do the turning with two people—one to lift and one to place the pillows. However, I wanted to give Mom a chance to rest.

My dad groaned a bit when I turned him, especially with the forceful hand heel pushing on his back. It was a first sign of pain. However, once the turning was over, he seemed perfectly comfortable again. I held off on the morphine.

After putting the head of the bed back up, I gave his mouth a good suctioning and administered two drops of atropine under his tongue. It was easy to do. Dad looked back at me as I screwed the cap back on the medicine bottle. Perhaps it was just my imagination, but the look on his face seemed to say: *What was that for?*

"Atropine," I said showing him the bottle. "Dries up mouth secretions. So you won't choke or cough as much."

I pulled the blankets up over his chest and sat back down in the blue armchair. "Clair de Lune" was playing on the radio. My dad closed his eyes, and soon he was asleep again, even snoring a little. *Good.* Things were going reasonably well. He was home. He was sleeping. He was comfortable. He was not suffering. Nevertheless, I couldn't help but feel a deep sadness. My dad was never going to get out of that bed. He was never going to get up and go feed his koi. He was never going to do another backyard project. He was never going to see his ranch in Mariposa again. This is where he was going die.

115

I went out to the living room to see how my mom was doing. She was watching a black-and-white movie with Jimmy Stewart. I asked her if she wanted something to eat. She said no.

"He seems comfortable," I said. "He's sleeping. I think he's tired. I'll bet he didn't get much sleep at the hospital."

Mom stared at the TV. She said nothing.

"You okay?" I asked after a moment.

"No, not really," she replied.

"What?"

"I thought it would be better when he got home. It's not."

"Yeah. I was thinking the same thing."

"It's too hard for me to go in there. I know I should. But, I don't like seeing him and knowing…. I don't know. That there's nothing we can do."

I sat down and put my arm around her. "It's okay," I said. "It's all right if you don't go in. I understand. He understands. I'll take care of things. You don't need to go in until you're ready."

Mom started to cry. "You're the strong one, now," she said. "It used to be your father. Now it's you."

I held her and felt her sobbing under my arms. To be perfectly honest, I didn't feel all that "strong" at that moment.

On the TV screen, Jimmy Stewart professed his love to a young, pretty woman wearing a fur coat.

*   *   *

I turned Dad at 7:00 and every two hours through the night. There was a little groaning with the turns. Other than that, he continued to appear comfortable. I suctioned out his

116

mouth with each turning and gave the atropine drops. After the wake-up and repositioning, he always fell quickly back to sleep.

After the 9:00 PM turn, Mom finally came into the room. She stood at the bed and held Dad's hand while I turned him. I was getting better at the turning job, and I didn't ask her for help. When I was finished, she sat in the blue chair and remained with Dad for half an hour. For the first time, he did not fall immediately back to sleep. He seemed to be aware that she was there with him, and he lay in bed just looking at her. She held his hand and silently stroked his forehead. It was so easy to see that she loved my father so much. Finally, Dad started to drift off to sleep. Mom whispered, "Good night, Sweetheart," and she kissed him on the cheek. Then, she stood up and headed off to the guest bedroom.

I went to my own bedroom, one room down the hall, and set the alarm for 11:00. I crawled into bed, leaving the doors to both my room and Dad's bedroom open. If I listened hard, I could just make out the sound of his breathing. I knew it was not going to be easy to sleep, knowing the alarm would go off in two short hours. I read a book for a little while, then turned off the light.

I nodded off for a short time, but I kept waking up and looking at the clock to see how much time was left before I had to get up. It reminded me of the days when I was a medical resident-in-training, and I had to sleep with a pager that would inevitably go off just as I drifted off to sleep.

As the night wore on, it became easier and easier to fall asleep between turnings. One o'clock. Three o'clock. After the five o'clock turning, I fell asleep as soon as my head hit the pillow, and I did not wake up until two hours later with the music blaring from my clock radio. 7:00 AM. The sun was streaming in the bedroom windows. The birds were chirping outside. A new day had begun.

XII. The Telling

Day 2.

At the 7:00 AM turning, I noticed his lips were starting to appear dry. No cracks or peeling skin, just a slightly dull appearance to the normal color, and the lip wrinkles seemed more prominent than usual. I moistened his lips with a lollipop sponge. His skin was starting to feel dry, too. When I suctioned him, his mouth secretions were getting thicker. The signs were there: early dehydration. He had to be feeling thirsty. Assuming he'd been getting IV fluids and NG feeds right up to the time of his hospital discharge yesterday, then he'd been about eighteen hours now without food or water. I checked his Foley bag—it was nearly full. He was still making urine at a good rate.

He was wide awake, turning his head from side to side. He didn't appear to be in any distress or discomfort. However, the sparkle in his eyes I'd seen yesterday was no longer there. Perhaps I was just imagining it, but the look on his face seemed somehow more serious and somber now.

He didn't groan or show any signs of pain when I turned him. I could tell he was getting used to the routine. After the turning, I pulled the bed sheet and the blanket up to his chest but left the comforter folded at the foot of the bed. With the sun streaming in through the windows, it was already a nice temperature in the room.

I went to the kitchen to make myself some breakfast. My mom's bedroom door was still shut. She would remain in bed till 11:00. I was going to bring my cereal and OJ back into the bedroom and sit with my dad, but I quickly realized this was a terrible idea. Could there be anything more rude and brainless

119

than to eat and drink in front of a hungry, thirsty man? I ate my breakfast alone in my dad's study. Out the window, the water in the koi pond sparkled as it flowed from the fountain and splashed down over the rocks. I watched the morning news on the TV for a few minutes. Then I went into the kitchen, washed my dishes, and headed back to the bedroom.

My dad was still awake, and I sat down in the blue chair next to the bed. After a minute, he started lifting his left arm. He touched the bed rail and let go, his arm dropping back to the bed. He repeated this movement—touching, letting go, touching, letting go. I got the impression he was trying to grab the rail in order to move or to sit up. Was he trying to get out of bed?

"Whatcha doing?" I asked, leaning into his line of vision.

He stopped his movements.

"You okay?"

He lay there, looking at me. I pressed the control button on the bed and brought his head up a little. I checked his mouth to see if he needed suctioning again. His secretions were minimal. I dipped a lollipop sponge in a glass of water and moistened his lips.

"Is that better?" I asked.

I tried to read his face for a clue. There was something about the lines of expression on the left side that made me feel uneasy. Once again, it was not a look of pain or discomfort. It was more a look of—I wasn't sure—perplexity, perhaps. Confusion?

Of course. Confusion. Could that be it? Then it dawned on me: he had no idea what was going on. Why should he? No one had told him. Specifically, no one had told him "the plan." Hospice, no feedings, no water, no antibiotics, no IVs…. *The plan.* I was sure no one at St. Mark's had told him. The

120

neurologist said he could understand what we said to him, but had anyone had the courtesy—or the courage—to tell him? How do you tell someone *that*? "Mr. Stookey, there's nothing more we can do for you. We're sending you home to die."

Did my dad even know the seriousness of his condition? We had talked about his condition and the prognosis at his bedside. Had he heard us? Had he understood?

He started reaching for the bedrail again. I couldn't help but think perhaps he was trying to get out of bed. I knew I had to at least try to tell him. Everything. The stroke, the prognosis, why we'd brought him home, what lay ahead. It was not right to let him lie there in ignorance as he became more hungry, more thirsty, more perplexed. It was going to be a hard, nearly an impossible "conversation." But I had to tell him.

I moved the chair closer to the bed and lowered the bedrail so there was nothing between my dad and me. I took hold of his hand and sat so he could see me.

"Dad," I said after a moment, squeezing his hand. "I just realized something. You're probably wondering what's going on. What's happening to you? Right? The neurologist at the hospital said you can understand, so…. So, I'm going to explain it to you. You deserve to know. Okay?" I squeezed his hand again.

My dad lay there looking back at me. It looked as though the lines on his face had moved into an expression of attention. Were the lines talking to me? *Yes, tell me everything. Yes.*

"You had a stroke, Dad. A very, very bad stroke. The part of your brain that controls your muscles got damaged. That's why you can't move. The part of your brain that controls speech and swallowing got damaged. That's why you can't talk or swallow."

I rubbed my dad's shoulder for a moment. "A stroke is a permanent thing. A part of the brain dies, and you never get it back. That means…. That means you're never going to walk again, Daddy. Never."

I hadn't called my father "Daddy" in over forty years.

"Since you can't swallow, you can't eat or drink. We could feed you and give you water by that tube in your nose. That's what the tube was supposed to be for. Or we could put a tube directly into you stomach." I gently poked my dad's belly. "Here. That's where the stomach tube would go. We could feed you that way. But…."

I paused. Another squeeze of the hand. The lines of attention on his face were still there.

"I don't think that's what you would want. Is it? *We* don't think that's what you want: me, Mom, Lori. Dr. Wilber, too. Use the tube, yes or no? Because even with the feeding tube, you still couldn't walk or swallow or talk. You still couldn't work in the yard. And the ranch, well…."

He looked at me, his eyes unblinking.

"I know you, Dad. I know you. I've seen your advanced directive: 'No heroic measures.' I know what you told Dr. Wilber about your wishes. I've even seen your 'Hemlock' file. Yup, I found it in the drawer in your desk, and I read it. You knew we would find it, didn't you? We can't give you hemlock, Dad. Or a pill or anything like that. It's illegal. We can't do that. It's just not an option."

What I'd said so far had been difficult. What came next was even harder.

"The people at the hospital were talking about sending you to a nursing home. I know you'd never want that. You told Dr. Wilber no nursing home, but I didn't need him to tell me that. If we took you to a nursing home, you'd die by inches there. Like your mom. But, we're not going to let that happen. No nursing home. Never. No way."

I sat there holding Dad's hand. Did he understand? I will never know for sure. There was a long moment of silence. A couple of times, I stated to speak but stopped. I couldn't bring myself to say the final words I needed to say.

"We have drugs to make everything easier," I finally said, without stating what "everything" was. "We have morphine for pain, and we have Ativan—it's a sedative. I'm going to be with you the whole time. The whole time. But we're not going to use the tube, Daddy." I touched his nose where the tube went in. "Okay? That's the plan. We're not going to use the tube because I don't think you want us to. Everything I know about you tells me that. I wish you could talk and tell me I'm right. But you can't, and that's okay. Because I already know. You don't need to tell me. I know."

Yes, I could have been clearer and more direct in what I was telling him. I'd done the best I could do. Dad was a smart man. If he could understand the way I thought he could—the way the neurologist said he could—then he knew what I was trying so hard to tell him.

I looked at his face for a reaction. Anything. But he never gave any gesture or sign. The expression on his face did not change. The days that followed might have been easier had he given an indication he understood and he agreed. The one thing that was different was that he was no longer reaching for the bedrail. He was no longer moving at all. He just lay there looking at me, his eyes never turning away from mine.

*   *   *

Later in the morning, my parents' cat came into the

123

bedroom, meowing. She—the little, white Persian—was hungry, no doubt. She was used to being fed at a much earlier hour. Dad had now fallen asleep, for which I was thankful. He looked peaceful. I picked up the little cat and held her on my lap as I watched the slow rise and fall of my dad's chest. After a few minutes, I tiptoed out of the room, carrying the cat out to the pantry. I poured out some cat food.

Taking a fifteen-minute break from the bedroom, I sat down on the back porch steps with a cup of coffee. The sound of a lawn mower came from the neighbor's backyard. Across the wall, I could see another neighbor riding an exercise bike in the upper story window of his house. The neighbors, the world, were proceeding forward with their day as usual. The only thing different was my father was not up and about with them. He was not in the backyard fishing leaves out of the koi pond or giving bits of sliced apple to his desert turtles. Instead, he was lying in a hospital bed in his bedroom, dying.

I finished my coffee, took a shower, and got dressed for the day.

XIII. Morphine

At 11:00 AM it was turning time again. Dad was awake, and, somewhat to my dismay, he was reaching for the bar again. In addition, there was a hint of a grimace on his face: the left corner of his mouth was turned slightly down, and his lower lip protruded just a little. His lips looked drier than they'd looked two hours ago, and I immediately reached for a lollipop sponge. Moistening his lips, I noticed he was breathing a little fast. Using my watch, I measured his breathing rate: twenty-two breaths per minute—a bit faster than the normal sixteen breaths per minute I'd measured yesterday.

"You okay, Dad?" I asked. "Are you in pain?" He looked at me, the grimace still there.

I decided to give him his first dose of morphine. Although I couldn't tell what—if anything—might be bothering him, he looked uncomfortable. I went to the kitchen, got the "Comfort Kit" from the refrigerator, and returned to the bedroom. Taking out the morphine bottle, I measure out five milligrams on the dropper—the dose for mild pain—and administered the dose under his tongue. He seemed a bit agitated as well (that repeated reaching for the rail); consequently, I gave him a dose of Ativan, half a milligram, the minimum dose.

After the meds, I turned him. He groaned a little as I got him settled back down on the pillows. I propped his legs up with additional pillows and moistened his lips again.

"Better?" I said stepping back.

But the grimace was still there. Moreover, within a short time, he started reaching for the bed rail again. *Why was he doing that?* Not knowing what else to do, I sat down in the chair, took hold of his hand in order to stop the reaching, and waited for the morphine and the Ativan to take effect.

While I waited, Mom emerged from her bedroom. I could see her from where I was sitting. The door opened, and she walked out looking a mess. She was usually quite attentive to her appearance and rarely presented herself in the morning without at least combing her hair. Not this morning. She came out of her room disheveled, wearing an untied bathrobe, and went straight to the bathroom. She didn't even notice me sitting there in the bedroom with Dad. I heard the toilet flush, and then I heard her walk out to the living room. She hadn't even bothered to come and look in on us.

Leaving Dad alone for a moment, I went out to the living room to see if she was okay. She was lying on the couch, an afghan comforter pulled up to her neck.

"You all right?" I asked.

"Oh—" she said, sounding a little startled. She looked at me as if she were going to say something, but remained silent.

"Do you want some tea or something?" I asked.

"No."

"Earl Grey?"

"No."

"You need to eat something. You hardly ate yesterday."

"Well…. Some tea, then."

"Something to eat. Toast?"

"No. Just tea."

"Are you going in? To see him?"

It was some time before she answered. "I'll drink my tea first," she said.

"You can sit with him," I said. "There's the blue chair by the bed. You could read. Watch TV. I'll bring the kitchen TV in and set it up."

126

"No. I don't want the TV. I'll go in in a little while."

"Want a banana?"

"Just the tea."

I went to the kitchen and made the tea. I also made some toast. It couldn't hurt to put a little food in front of her. I brought the tea and toast back into the living room and sat down.

"He seems a tiny bit agitated this morning," I said. "I gave him some medicine to help him relax."

My mom sipped her tea but said nothing. As expected, she didn't eat the toast. After she finished her tea, we went in together to see Dad. He was wide awake, dashing my hopes that the morphine and the Ativan might put him out for a few hours. And he was still doing that reaching, over and over. Mom sat down in the blue chair.

There was another chair in the room, a loveseat against the far wall. I went over and sat down. Mom gazed silently at Dad and held his hand. The radio played classical music against the sound of the waterfall and the chirping birds.

After five minutes, I heard Mom sniffing, and I saw she was crying. I got up and gave her a Kleenex.

"I'm going to go back to the living room now," she said, dabbing her eyes. "Okay?"

"Of course," I said. "I'll stay here. You go. I'll stay with him."

She left, and I heard the TV turn on in the living room. Admittedly, I'd envisioned things differently. I'd imagined she would have kept a constant vigil in the room, sitting with Dad, perhaps reading or watching TV there. I'd even considered setting up a second bed in the room so she could sleep with him. But this was not to be. It was not a sign, though, that she didn't love my father. Not at all. In fact, just the opposite.

127

Dad remained awake for much of the rest of the day, and he continued to appear restless—reaching for the rail, turning his head, looking around the room. Looking for what? I gave him more morphine and Ativan, but, to my surprise, it didn't seem to make much difference. I even doubled the dose in the afternoon, yet he remained restless. I knew he had to be thirsty. He'd now been two full days without water. His skin was looking drier, and the color of the urine in the Foley bag was darker. He was still making urine but at a diminishing rate.

I tried putting a moistened washcloth on his forehead, and I turned on the table fan next to his bed. I moistened his lips several times an hour. Despite these measures, the restlessness continued. Nothing seemed to help. No water for forty-eight hours. As hard as it was for me to think about it, I feared the reaching for the rail might be a sign of agitation due to thirst. He wanted water.

*   *   *

Marcia stopped by at 4:00. I told her about my dad's apparent agitation. She said this was common at this stage—he was still fully conscious, but he might be feeling some restlessness from being "so long in bed." She reviewed the doses of morphine and Ativan I'd been giving.

"Good!" she said. She seemed pleased. "Most people are afraid to give more than the minimal dose. You moved right up to the higher doses. Nice."

We went into the bedroom together. Dad was awake, his eyes open and pointed toward the bed rail, and he was still reaching for the rail. Marcia went to the bedside and took his hand.

"Hey, Bill, it's Marcia." She looked him over, checking his

skin, looking into his mouth, and feeling his forehead for signs of a fever.

We turned him together—I lifted while Marcia stuffed the pillows. After the turning, he seemed more comfortable. There was no more reaching. Maybe his reaching was an attempt to roll over in bed. I imagined how uncomfortable it must be to want to change position and to be unable to do so.

Marcia emptied the Foley bag. "His urine output is really going to drop off over the next twenty-four hours," she said to me in the bathroom where Dad couldn't hear. "His kidneys will start to shut down over the next couple days."

Back at the bedside, she gave Dad an additional dose of morphine and Ativan even though he looked pretty comfortable now. She gave the highest dose of morphine, twenty milligrams. "It'll help him sleep," she said. "Remember, eight years doing hospice, and I haven't seen anyone give an overdose yet."

I was tempted to say, *That's too bad; perhaps it would be the kindest thing.* But I held back.

After the morphine and Ativan, we went into the living room and talked to my mom. She was still sitting on the couch. Marcia said Dad seemed "very comfortable." I don't think this was quite true, but I forgave her, knowing she was only trying to reassure Mom. She told us someone named Arnold, the hospice attendant, would be by tomorrow morning to bathe my dad, shave him, and wash his hair.

After talking to my mom, Marcia and I went back to check on Dad one more time. He was asleep. Lying there on his side, his breathing was soft and even. He looked as peaceful as a sleeping baby.

"Fantastic," I said with a sigh of relief.

Marcia tiptoed to the bedside and whispered to my dad,

so as not to wake him: "See you tomorrow, Bill. Sleep well."

I walked her to the door.

"Sorry I was a little late today," she said. "I had a patient pass away this morning. Nothing unexpected. Cancer."

"You have a hard job," I said.

"Oh—there's a lot of sadness, yes, but there's also a lot of satisfaction. I'll tell you one thing: you see people at their most real, working hospice. All the phoniness, the games people play in regular life, the petty worries and squabbles—it all gets pushed aside. There's sadness but there's also honesty. I like honesty. Life is short. This job makes you appreciate that and to value the time we have. It also makes you appreciate family, friends, loved ones. Never take those relationships for granted. Anyway. Bye, Chris. See you tomorrow."

"See you tomorrow," I said.

"You're doing a good job. Keep an eye on your mom, though. If she doesn't want to go into the room, that's fine. But she really needs you right now. Spend some time with her, too."

"I will," I said. "I promise."

XIV. Hesitations

Day 3.

The next morning I woke up at 6:00, an hour before turning time. I got up and checked on Dad. He was still sleeping peacefully. I might have done an early turning had he been awake, but I decided to let him sleep. I tiptoed out of the room and headed for the kitchen, where I made myself some coffee. Sitting down at the desk in the study, I turned on the computer and spent the next half-hour Internet-researching the topic of dehydration. I goggled the phrase "death by dehydration," having no idea what I would find. The search turned up over fourteen million results.

In the medical world and the world of hospice, death by dehydration is known as "terminal dehydration." Looking over the first page of web links, I quickly saw that terminal dehydration, as a means of hastening death, is a controversial topic. There are two camps of thought. One camp—I'll call them the "pro-TD" camp—believes that terminal dehydration is a relatively painless and peaceful way to die; a "serene form of death" is the phrase they often use. The other camp—the "anti-TD" camp—claims just the opposite. They say death by dehydration is a cruel, brutal, and painful death.

Members of the first camp tend to be physicians, hospice workers, and death-with-dignity advocates. Members of the second camp are, in general, people with ties to religious organizations and right-to-life groups.

I explored the views of both camps. The anti-TD camp asserts that terminal dehydration is anything but "serene." According to an article posted by the Catholic Education Resource Center, death by dehydration leads to an "agonizing" death marked by pangs of thirst, cracked lips, nosebleeds (due to dry mucous membranes), and vomiting (due to a dried stomach lining). Another article by the Family Research Council described TD as "a gruesome form of death" where the tongue cracks and bleeds, the eyes sink into the orbits, and the skin peels off upon contact. Operation rescue, the Christian fundamentalist group, states death by dehydration is "one of the most horrible ways to die." Quoting their website: "Just try going for one day without ANY food or liquids—and see how you feel. You won't like it!"

On the other hand, the pro-TD camp claims that terminal dehydration is neither agonizing nor cruel. As dehydration sets in, they say, the body releases certain chemicals ("esters" and "ketones") that have the effect of dulling the senses. These chemicals act like an anesthetic. As a result, patients dying of dehydration feel little pain, and they often require less pain medication and sedation than patients receiving fluids via stomach tubes and IVs. Symptoms of dehydration, such as dry mouth, can be alleviated by wetting the lips and the tongue and by giving ice chips. One article described a poll of hospice nurses who ranked death experiences on a scale of 1 (the most undesirable death) to 10 (the most comfortable death). They gave terminal dehydration an 8.

A *Los Angeles Times* article quoted a Dr. Ira Byock, director of palliative medicine at Dartmouth Medical Center, as saying: "The cessation of eating and drinking is the dominant way mammals die. It is a very gentle way that nature has provided for animals to leave this life."

Of course, it's impossible to know what death by dehydration is really like. The fact of death precludes a retelling of the experience. I felt there were problems with both the pro- and anti-TD viewpoints. The anti-TD camp seemed to be arguing largely from emotion with arguments focusing on impassioned visuals like sunken eyes and cracked lips. It seemed ironic to me that the religiously-affiliated groups should argue so fervently in favor of sustaining terminally ill patients by artificial means (such as NG tubes and IVs). They seemed to be arguing for human over divine intervention. Why wasn't the religious community more philosophically sympathetic to the idea of stopping the tube feeds and the IVs and leaving matters in the hands of God?

At the same time, I wasn't so sure I bought Ira Byock's idea that "nature" had provided a "gentle" way for people and animals to die. Nature is blind to human and animal suffering, and nature can be extremely cruel. The simple fact that mammals commonly die naturally of dehydration does not necessarily mean the process is "gentle."

I decided the truth probably lay somewhere between the extremes of the two camps. In a conscious patient, like my dad, it seemed there would have to be some period of time marked by a sensation of thirst, including severe thirst, and this would have to be uncomfortable. I tried to think of a time when I had been extremely thirsty without access to water, but I could think of no such experience in my own life. So, I tried to *imagine* the sensation of extreme thirst, with every cell of my body screaming for a sip of water. I had to say, my imaginings were not very pleasant.

At the same time, I gave a lot of credence to the observations of hospice nurses. These were the people on the front line, the people who saw death on a regular basis, and they knew the difference between a "good death" and a "bad death." Most of these nurses had rated terminal dehydration as a relatively good death. Moreover, I knew from my own work as a doctor that there were far more gruesome ways to die. The poll of hospice workers did not state the "*least* desirable" way to die, but I thought about what it might be: a slow withering away in some ICU, strapped down with restraints in a bed, alone, tethered to a respirator, tubes inserted in various orifices, needles in both arms.

I had to believe that terminal dehydration was at least better than death by a thousand assaults in the ICU. Yet this is how many people die these days.

I finished my coffee and turned off the computer.

*   *   *

At 7:00 AM, I went back into the bedroom to turn Dad. Much to my surprise, I found him awake and all twisted in bed. Just an hour ago, he had been sleeping peacefully. Now, his left leg had fallen off the pillow used to prop it up. His head had slid off his pillows, and he was lying with his neck awkwardly flexed forward. His left arm was extended out through the bedrails, and he was making circular movements with his hand. A line of saliva ran from the corner of his mouth to his ear. He looked awful—uncomfortable, breathing hard, twisted, completely unable to right himself.

"Hey," I said, stepping quickly to the bedside, "what happened!" I moved his arm in through the rails, rolled him onto his back, and put his head back squarely on the pillow. With a moistened washcloth, I wiped off his face.

I reassessed him now that he was straightened out, but he *still* looked uncomfortable. His breathing remained rapid, and there was a look of discomfort on his face. Was it pain? Was it thirst? His lips now looked very dry: there was no cracking or bleeding, but the skin was shriveled and dotted with light-colored flecks. I knew that this was the point at which he'd probably be feeling thirst at its keenest—two days without water but not yet at the stage where the "sedating ketones and esters" had built up in his blood. In other words, thirsty but still fully conscious.

I reached for the morphine and dropped twenty milligrams under his tongue, and I followed this with a dose of Ativan. After the drugs, I ran a moistened sponge lollipop over his lips and inside his mouth.

But, there was still no change in the expression on his face. What was that look? Anguish? Confusion? Dread? I hated it, whatever it was. I couldn't help but remember the expression of joy we'd seen on his face when he'd come home from the hospital two days ago. That look was entirely gone now.

After half an hour, he seemed to calm down a little. His breathing slowed; the look of discomfort began to fade. I assumed the drugs were kicking in. He closed his eyes. To my great relief, he fell back to sleep.

*   *   *

At 9:00 AM, Arnold, the home health aide, arrived. He was a pleasant, middle-aged Filipino man. I took him into the bedroom and introduced him to Dad, who was awake but sleepy. I asked Arnold what I needed to do to help.

"Nothing," he said. "Take a break, Chris. Let me take over for a little while."

"It's time for his nine o'clock turning," I said.

"No problem, I'll turn him. You go ahead, take a break."

I took Arnold up on his offer. I made myself another cup of coffee and took it out to the backyard. It was a beautiful, sunny morning, and I sat down in the patio area. A squirrel scampered across the top of the south wall; a robin sang in the cottonwood above the trellis. Shortly after I sat down, the cat came over and jumped up into my lap. I rubbed her back, and she rolled over on her side, purring. I think she missed the daily attention she was used to getting from Mom and Dad. I scratched her neck as we both soaked up the sun filtering down through the cottonwood.

It was well past 10:00 when Arnold came out to tell me he was finished. "Okay, Chris," he said. "All done. I shaved your dad, gave him a sponge bath, washed his hair. He looks good. Just one problem I can see: he's developing a little redness on the tailbone area."

"Redness?" I said. I was surprised; I hadn't noticed any redness. "Do you mean a bed sore?"

"It could be the very start of one. But I think we can nip it in the bud if we're careful."

Careful? But I *had* been careful. I'd been meticulously careful. "I've been turning him every two hours," I said. "On the clock."

"I know. The problem is there's still a spot that's getting some pressure. He has a little strength in his left arm and leg, and he moves around just enough to slide off the pillows. Then he can't lift himself up to shift the weight off the pressure area."

What Arnold said made sense. "Yeah. I found him this morning hanging halfway out the rails. Damn, that's the one thing I want to avoid: bedsores."

"It's not bad, Chris. We'll keep a close eye on it. I'll let Marcia know."

I walked Arnold to the door and thanked him for coming out. I felt terrible about the bedsore. Dad feared bedsores; they were the one of the things he always mentioned when he

136

talked about the horrible way his mother had died. I wanted to avoid bedsores at all costs—but now, just two days after coming home, there were the first signs of one.

"Damn!" I said out loud walking back to the bedroom. I felt as though I had let my dad down.

I went back into the bedroom, and there was Dad propped up on his side, looking much better now. Arnold had done a fantastic job. He'd given him a close, clean shave, and his face looked so smooth and fresh. His hair was shiny clean, too, and neatly combed. My dad still had a full head of hair, and, although he was almost completely gray now, his hair retained a healthful vigor with its natural waviness and sheen. With the shave and the combed hair, I couldn't help but note that my dad, who'd been quite handsome in his youth, was still a good-looking man.

"You look great!" I said, sitting down in the blue chair. I noticed Arnold had even trimmed and cleaned my dad's fingernails. I was impressed. Arnold had done a superb job.

I searched Dad's face for that "look" I'd noticed earlier, the look of discomfort. To my great relief, it was no longer there. I smiled. Perhaps it was the bathing that had him feeling better. Perhaps it was the morphine and Ativan I'd given just before Arnold arrived. Perhaps it was getting the weight off the sore area on his back.

I had to take a look for myself. I wanted to see the bedsore. I went around to the other side of the bed, lowered the bedrail, lifted the covers, and gently pulled down the fresh pair of diapers Arnold had put on. At the low, middle part of Dad's back, just above the buttocks, the skin was indeed red and a little raw-looking. Arnold had applied some powder to the red area, which was perhaps two inches round in diameter. The skin was still intact; there was no ulcer.

At the same time, I knew the red area must be associated with some pain. In fact, bedsores are the most painful in the early stages, when the skin is raw but still intact. The deeper bedsores—the ones that eat through the skin down to muscle and even to bone—they look much worse, but they're actually less painful because the skin and the sensitive nerve endings have been destroyed.

I wondered if the signs of distress I'd observed earlier might have been due to that raw area. Maybe that's why I'd found him all twisted in bed; with what little strength he had, he'd been trying to relieve the pressure on his lower back.

When Mom woke up, I pulled her into the bedroom. Arnold had done such a good job, I wanted her to see Dad looking so neat and fresh.

"Have a look," I said, leading her into the room.

I could see from the look on Mom's face that she, too, was impressed.

"Doesn't he look good?" I said.

"Yes," she said, sitting down in the blue chair. "You've given him a shave."

"No, Arnold, the health aide, did it. He was here a little while ago."

"His hair looks so nice." Mom smiled. "I was always jealous of his hair—he has the nice hair, not me." She sat in silence looking at Dad. I could see it made her happy to see him looking so fresh and clean. However, after a minute, the smile on her face faded away, and she became quiet.

"It's almost harder this way," she said after a minute, choking a little on her words. "For a minute, I…."

I knew what she was going to say. For a minute, she had forgotten.

"I know," I said.

138

My mom stood up. "I'll go to the living room now."

"I'll bring you some toast and fresh fruit. Maybe some eggs?"

"Nothing right now. Maybe some tea in a little while."

"No. You're going to eat something, Mom."

"Well, some toast, then. Just a slice."

* * *

At 2:00, my sister arrived. I took her into the bedroom, and she sat with Dad for half an hour. He was awake. He'd only slept for a couple of hours in the morning. Since then, he'd been awake and a little restless. I'd given him more morphine and Ativan.

I left Lori alone with my dad and went to the living room to sit with Mom. When Lori came out and sat down with us, she had a troubled look on her face. She started to speak, but stopped.

"What?" I asked.

"I don't know," Lori said. "It's just…. I think—the way we're not doing anything…."

"Not doing anything?" I said.

"Not feeding him. No water. Dr. Wilber said he would get pneumonia, and that that was…a kind way to go."

"Yes," I said.

"Well…. Then, why can't we just give him some water? If he's going to die of pneumonia anyway, at least he doesn't have to die of thirst, too."

"So you're saying, use the feeding tube," I said. "Feed him, give him water."

"Water, at least."

"But if we do that," I said, "it might just prolong things."

139

"And that's bad?" Lori said. "Remember, we left that as an option."

"It's just…. I don't think that's what he wants," I said.

My sister didn't respond. I have to say, I understood the way she felt. It *was* hard to just sit by and watch him die. It was excruciatingly hard. Apparently for my sister, it had become too hard.

Mom had remained silent while Lori and I talked. She lay on the couch, looking down at her hands, fiddling with the threads of her afghan.

"I know what you're saying, Lori, but I don't think we should change course," I said. "It's hard for me, too, believe me. But I think this is what Dad wants—what we're doing now. If he could talk, he'd probably ask us to give him hemlock. The last thing he'd want would be for us to drag everything out. That's what I think. I'm just one vote out of three, though."

My sister and my mom remained silent.

"You know what?" I said. "I think you two should talk about it, just the two of you. I'll get out of the way." I stood up. "I'm going to step out, leave you two to talk. Okay?"

Lori nodded. "Okay," she said.

I started to walk out. Then I stopped and turned back. "Just so you know," I said, "he's starting to get a bedsore."

"He is?" Mom said.

"Yeah. On his lower back. It's a small one, and we're taking care of it. But he moves around a little bit, and he keeps sliding off his pillows. It's hard to keep the pressure off that area."

Mom frowned but said nothing more.

"Just so you know," I said.

I walked out of the living room, leaving them alone. So

140

far, I had always been present for our family discussions. But now I wanted Lori and Mom to reach their own decision. Whatever they decided, I would go with that. If they wanted to give Dad water, fine. Lori was right—if we gave him water, eventually he would get pneumonia from aspirating his mouth secretions. Death by pneumonia. Perhaps it would be a better way to go.

I went out to the backyard and sat down next to the koi pond. I thought about what might happen if we gave Dad water. He would almost certainly live longer. Weeks? Possibly even months, if we gave him food as well. Of course, we would keep him at home; there was no question about that. We would hire someone to help us out. I knew hospice could provide an attendant; someone like Arnold would be perfect. I resigned myself to accept whatever decision my mom and Lori reached.

After about ten minutes, I went back to the living room. Mom was there alone.

"Where's Lori?" I asked.

"She left. She had to go home."

"So?" I said sitting down on the sofa next to Mom. "Do we start giving him water? Did you decide?"

Mom was silent for some time. Then, finally, she said: "No."

"No? Meaning 'no you haven't decided' or 'no water?'"

My mom turned away from me without answering and looked out the living room window. The mailman had just delivered the mail to our porch, and he was walking out the driveway toward the house next door. You could hear the rattle of the mail truck's engine at the curb.

Then, still looking blankly out the window, my mom said, her voice barely audible: "Water. I mean, no water."

141

XV. The Hardest Day

Day 4.

My alarm sounded at 7:00 AM. When I walked into the bedroom, I once again found Dad twisted in bed. His head was off his pillow, and his face was tilted backwards as though he were trying to look—upside-down—out the windows into the backyard. His left leg stuck out through the bedrail bars and hung off the bed. His left arm was extended up in the air propped up against the bedrail. He'd slid off all his body pillows, and he was completely uncovered, lying flat on his back.

Just looking at him, I could see his weight was concentrated on his lower back—exactly on the area of the pressure sore. It was as though this was his center of gravity, and, no matter how he moved or twisted, the laws of physics brought his weight inevitably down on precisely this spot.

Even more troubling than his awkward position, however, was that he appeared to be in pain. There was a blatant grimace on his face, and beads of perspiration dotted his forehead. He was breathing rapidly, even making a slight grunting sound with each exhalation. In short, he looked awful. I was horror-struck.

I rushed over to the bedside. "What are you doing?" I asked sharply, as though his awkward position in bed were something intentional and entirely his fault.

I used the bed controls and immediately lowered his head and legs until the bed was flat. Then, pulling his head and his legs to the center of the bed, I straightened him out. He moaned as I moved him. I rolled him on his side—more moaning—and immediately began stuffing pillows underneath

142

in order to get the weight off his lower back. Once I had him propped up, I checked the red area on his back. "*Damn*," I said under my breath. It was redder than yesterday, and larger. Whereas twelve hours ago the sore had been a light pinkish color, it was now an angry brick red. The skin still appeared intact; there were no blisters or ulcers. However, I noticed that in the center of the red area, there was a slight seepage of a clear fluid. The skin was one step away from blister formation, and it looked painful. Very painful.

Morphine, morphine. I gave him a full twenty milligrams, the maximum dose, and chased it down with two milligrams of Ativan (again, the maximum).

While I waited for the drugs to kick in, I moistened Dad's lips and toweled his face. I checked the urine in his Foley bag. There were only about 100 ccs in the bag since Arnold had emptied it yesterday. Over the last twenty hours, my dad had only produced three ounces of urine. Less than half a cup. The urine was a dark, caramel color. He had been nearly seventy-two hours without water now. Soon his kidneys would start to shut down altogether. It was the body's natural response to extreme dehydration.

I moistened his lips a second time. Then I sat down in the blue chair and waited.

Twenty minutes later, he still seemed distressed and in pain. The grimace was still there, the breathing still fast. There were occasional groans and moans. The morphine and Ativan should have taken effect by now. I assumed the cause of his distress was a combination of the painful sore on his lower back and thirst. I decided to give him another ten milligrams of morphine and another milligram of Ativan.

Yes, I was now stepping outside the parameters for the administration of these drugs—the maximum morphine dose was supposed to be twenty milligrams every two hours. I didn't care. Dad was in pain. I was not concerned about an overdose. The previous dose of morphine seemed to have had no effect at all. I gave the extra medication and, once again, sat down and waited.

After another twenty minutes, there was not much change. Despite the extra morphine and moistening his lips every ten minutes, he was still grimacing, still breathing fast. He was moving his left arm and leg; I had to keep putting his left leg back up on the pillows.

Why wasn't the morphine working better? I knew many people experienced a "high" when they received large doses of morphine, but some people experienced the opposite effect: hallucinations, a frightening loss of control, feelings of panic. It's called a "dysphoric reaction." Was this happening to Dad?

My greater suspicion, however, was that the real problem was that raw area on his back. Even though the pressure was now off the sore, I knew it must still be painful. It was like a second-degree burn, and that burn was going to continue to hurt even without the pressure. It was just a matter of giving enough pain medication, I thought.

So I made the decision. Morphine. More morphine. Another ten milligrams.

I sat, and I waited.

Half an hour later: *still no change*. Maybe he was a little calmer, but I was not satisfied. He was still awake. Still breathing fast. Still restless. Still moving his arm and leg. For an hour and a half now—forty milligrams of morphine, four of Ativan—I'd made little progress. The whole goal was to make him as comfortable as possible, and we weren't there yet. I reached for the drug bottle again, and I sucked twenty milligrams of morphine into the dropper. If I gave another maximal dose of morphine, I would be giving three times the recommended dose in under two hours. I didn't care. I pushed the dropper tip into his mouth and squirted another twenty milligrams under his tongue. I chased this with another two milligrams of Ativan.

I sat back down in the blue chair. And waited.

*   *   *

At nine o'clock the doorbell rang. It was Marty Lewis, my dad's best friend. A civil engineer in his late fifties, Marty had worked for my dad's engineering firm until Dad's forced resignation. After that, Marty left Willdan and went to work for another engineering firm. He and Dad had remained close. Marty stopped by the house regularly; they went out for drinks every week or two, and they even bought some real estate together. Now, Marty had come by the house to pay his respects.

"Hi, Chris," he said, standing at the door, dressed casually in slacks and a polo shirt. "I came by to see your dad. How's he doing?"

"Marty, hi," I said. "Come in. He's, uh—a little restless this morning. I've been giving him morphine."

"Oh, is it a bad time to visit?"

"No, no. He's in the bedroom. He'd love to see you."

We stepped into the living room and talked for a moment. Mom was still in bed. Marty said he'd visited Dad in the hospital, and he knew about the stroke and the seriousness of his condition. He did not, however, know about "the plan." Thus, before taking him into the bedroom, I brought Marty up to date: "Just so you understand—" I hesitated and looked him in the eyes. "We're not giving him any food or water." Marty

145

nodded somberly. I didn't need to explain any further. He understood, and he did not seem surprised by what I had just told him.

"As you'll see," I said, "we've left the NG tube in, but we're…not planning to use it."

I led Marty into the bedroom. Despite the multiple doses of morphine and Ativan, Dad was still awake. He was still reaching with his arm, but not so much now—that was at least a small improvement.

"Hey, Dad, look who's here," I said. "Marty!"

Marty stepped to the side of the bed. "Hi, Bill," he said in a solemn tone. To his credit, Marty did not appear to be startled by or even uncomfortable with Dad's appearance. The look on Marty's face was simply one of friendship and sympathy.

"I'm going to let you sit with him for a while if that's all right," I whispered. "It'll give me a chance to have a quick breakfast and a cup of coffee."

"Sure, Chris. Go ahead. Bill and I will have a visit, sure."

Out in the kitchen, I made a bowl of cereal and cup of black coffee. I sat down at the kitchen table. It was good to be out of the bedroom for a little while.

Marty stayed with Dad for twenty minutes. He came out to the kitchen while I was washing my cereal bowl and coffee cup.

"Thanks, Chris—for letting me stop by and the visit."

"No, thank *you*. I appreciate it, and I know my dad does, too."

"He looks.… Well, I'm glad I stopped by."

"Yeah. It's hard, Marty."

"How's your mom doing?"

"Not well. She spends most of the day in bed or in the

living room watching TV. She doesn't go in to see him much. It's just too much for her. It's hard for all of us."

"Chris…do you mind if I tell you a story? Something your dad once told me."

"Sure, of course."

"It might make you feel better about—what you're doing."

"Sure," I said. I gestured toward one of the kitchen chairs. Marty sat down. "Coffee?" I asked.

"No, I have to get to work. I'll make it quick."

I sat down at the table across from Marty.

"Do you remember when your dad had his heart attack?" he began. "When was it? Twenty years ago?"

"Yeah, about that," I said.

"That heart attack took your dad completely by surprise. Of course, it shouldn't have—he smoked two packs of cigarettes a day."

"Three," I said.

"Yeah, literally a chain smoker. Anyway, your dad thought he was somehow immune to heart trouble. His parents both had healthy hearts. He was an active guy. At first, he didn't believe it when his doctors told him he'd had a heart attack. He was sure the chest pain had to be lung cancer."

"Sounds like my dad," I said.

"Yeah. He even went and got a second opinion. I remember that. But the second opinion was the same as the first: 'You had a heart attack, Buddy.'"

I chuckled. "I can just hear my dad saying, 'No, you're wrong, Doctor.'"

Marty also laughed. "Yep. But, eventually, he accepted it. He accepted that he had a bad ticker. And one day over coffee—I don't know where we were, Denny's or some

147

place—one day over coffee, he said something very interesting."

"What?"

"He told me having a heart attack—and I quote—having a heart attack was 'the best thing that ever happened' to him."

"How's that, the best thing?"

"I didn't get it either, at first, but he explained. He said, 'Now that I've had a heart attack, the odds are I'll die of another one, another heart attack.' And he was happy about that. I mean, seriously happy. He figured it was a better way to go than to die of cancer. As a matter of fact, he told me his dream scenario of how he wanted to die."

"Dream scenario?"

"Yeah. He said he hoped that, one day, he'd be out bailing hay to his cows up at the ranch, and suddenly he'd just drop dead of a coronary. Wham. Here one minute, gone the next. He joked about how it might take a day or two for someone to find him out there in the barnyard, his cows mooing and trying to wake him up so they'd get fed. 'Who cares how long I'm lying there?' he said. 'My cows can stomp on me and crap on me. What do I care? I'll be dead.'"

"That's a bit macabre," I said.

"Yeah. But, I swear, the thought made your dad happy. Sudden and quick. Like being struck by lightening. Poof!" Marty snapped his fingers.

"My dad had a file in his desk drawer," I said. "It's labeled 'Hemlock.' It's about end-of-life stuff. He didn't want any heroics to keep him alive."

"To be brutally honest," Marty said, "I think right now he would prefer that bolt of lightening."

"Or a slug of hemlock," I said. A thought occurred to me. Maybe *that's* what he was reaching for. Hemlock.

148

"What?" Marty asked, seeing that I was suddenly lost in thought.

"Oh…nothing," I said. "Nothing. Thanks for the story. It helps. It helps because…." I paused.

"Because it shows you that you're doing the right thing," Marty said finishing my sentence.

*   *   *

After Marty left, I went back to the bedroom. Dad was still awake. He was still moving his left arm—reaching. He was still breathing fast. He still seemed uncomfortable. Why? Bedsore? Hunger? Thirst?

I gave him another dose of morphine. Twenty milligrams.

As I sat at the bedside, hoping the latest morphine dose would turn the tide, I found myself feeling frustrated. Frustrated and even angry. Why did he have to suffer at all? More to the point, why did he have to die like this? Slowly and possibly in pain? Couldn't we do better? Couldn't we knock him out, render him unconscious? Some sort of general anesthesia?

Or, why not give him what he really wanted? Hemlock. Or its modern-day equivalent. Oh yes, euthanasia was not permitted in California, but the crazy thing is, what we were doing right now to my dad *was* euthanasia. This *was* mercy killing. We were killing him just as surely as if we were giving him hemlock or cyanide or potassium chloride. The only difference was, we were killing him slowly. Dehydration was the hemlock we offered. Could we not offer a more humane path to death? Give him something faster acting? An overdose with a barbiturate, that would do the job—*gently*—in a matter of minutes. Terminal dehydration took five or six days. Or a week. Or longer. Yet, the end result would be the same: death.

We were more gentle and rational with our family pets. No one would ever use dehydration as a means to put down the family dog. No one would ever use starvation as a way to end the life of the family cat. It would be considered barbaric. Yet this is what we were doing to my father. He, who wanted hemlock. It was his body, his life—shouldn't it be *his* death?

Dad groaned a little. He reached out his left arm.

I will be honest, the thought occurred to me: Doing what I believed Dad wished I would do. I had the Ativan, and I had the morphine. Why not empty the entire bottle of each into his mouth? Would it be enough? I wasn't sure. I picked up the bottle of morphine. It contained a total of thirty milliliters, twenty milligrams of morphine per milliliters. Six hundred milligrams total (minus what we'd already used). Of course, it would be homicide if it worked.

And there were "practical" considerations. Marcia and hospice were monitoring the drugs I would administer. Frankly, I don't know how Marcia would react if I did it. Professionally, she couldn't approve of such an act—I knew that. Yet how strongly would she disapprove if Dad were to die sooner than expected, and the morphine bottle turned up empty?

But it wasn't just Marcia who was monitoring the drugs. There was the physician who was supervising her. I could claim I'd misunderstood the amount of drug I was supposed to administer. Unfortunately, it would be harder for me, a physician, to plead ignorance.

Still, in that moment of anger and frustration, I considered it.

But…. I didn't do it. I suppose I lacked the courage. Instead of an overdose with morphine, I moistened my dad's lips. I wiped his face with a damp washcloth. I suctioned a small amount of saliva from his mouth. All the while, he kept looking at me with that look in his eyes. That look of perplexity. That look that seemed to say: *Why are you doing this to me, Son? Please. Help me. Where is my hemlock?*

*   *   *

I sat the rest of the morning into the afternoon with him. I gave him the maximum dose of morphine once an hour. And yet, he continued to appear uncomfortable. The morphine didn't seem to be helping that much. I could give him twenty milligrams or nothing at all—it didn't seem to make much of a difference.

At three o'clock, Marcia arrived. I met her at the door and told her about how Dad had been in discomfort all day long. I told her that the bedsore was looking worse and that I'd been giving more morphine and Ativan than the instructions called for. Marcia remained calm as I told her this news. "Come on," she said, "let's go in and see him."

We went into the bedroom. He was breathing at a rate of thirty, and beads of perspiration dotted his forehead. Marcia looked over the log sheet, where I'd written down all doses of morphine and Ativan I'd given. I was afraid she was going to pounce on me for grossly exceeding the protocol. Her reaction was just the opposite.

"Whoa!" she said giving me a look of surprise. "Good for you! Very aggressive!"

And, then she proceeded to get even more aggressive. She picked up the morphine bottle and immediately gave Dad *forty* milligrams.

"If twenty isn't doing the job," she said, "we'll double it."

After giving the morphine, as well as a dose of Ativan, Marcia took a closer look at the sore on my dad's back. "Yes," she said. "It's redder. That's going to be painful."

"I've been turning him on schedule," I said, "but he keeps sliding off the pillows."

"Sometimes you do everything right, and you still get bed sores. They just can't be avoided."

Marcia gently cleaned the sore and applied some powder. We propped Dad up on pillows so there was absolutely no pressure on his lower back. Despite the repositioning and the double dose of morphine, the grimacing and the fast breathing continued without any sign of improvement.

Without hesitation, Marcia reached for the morphine and gave a second forty-milligram dose. She looked inside the bottle. "Where're getting low," she said. "I'll order another bottle."

And then she did a beautiful thing. With Dad lying on his back, propped up on his side, she went to the head of the bed on his left side. Facing him, she put her hand on his face, and she pressed her forehead against the side of his head. She began talking to him, her mouth right next to his ear. "We're going to take away the pain," she said in a confident yet soothing tone. "We're going to take it away. I'm going to stay right here until the pain is gone. I promise." She kept repeating this—"We're going to take the pain away"—while stroking his cheek and leaning her head against his. It was the perfect depiction of the compassionate nurse giving succor to a patient. It reminded me of a painting I'd once seen, a Civil War painting of a nurse giving comfort to a dying soldier.

Over and over: "It's okay, Bill. We're going to make the pain go away. We're going to take it away."

After the *four* doses—160 milligrams—of morphine, the

reaching finally stopped. The grimace was gone. My dad's breathing rate had come down to twenty. Actually, it was irregular now. He would breathe at a rate of twenty for a minute, then at a rate of ten. Back up to twenty; back down to ten. Marcia was not worried about the irregular breathing. She said it was a sign we'd gotten the dose of morphine about right.

She remained with him for another half an hour (she'd already been there an hour giving the doses of morphine). She wanted to be absolutely sure he was comfortable before she left. She moistened his lips; she talked to him; she stroked his cheek and held his hand.

Finally, he fell asleep.

We tiptoed out of the bedroom and went out to the living room. Marcia sat down with Mom. She opened her satchel and brought out a six-pack of Ensure, the nutritional drink. "I brought this for you," she said to Mom. "Ensure. Do you like vanilla? Betty?"

My mom gave a barely perceptible nod of her head.

"Good. I want you to drink two cans a day. Okay? Those are my orders." Marcia opened a can and poured the contents out in a glass. She handed the glass to Mom. "Bill is comfortable," she said. "He's sleeping now." She took hold of my mom's hand. "He's sleeping."

Marcia stayed and coaxed Mom to drink down her entire glass of Ensure. Then Marcia and I went back and checked on Dad one last time. He was still asleep, well positioned on his pillows. It was such a relief to see him looking truly comfortable for the first time since 7:00 this morning.

"I'll have another bottle of morphine delivered this evening," Marcia said. "Give forty milligrams at a time if you need to. He seems to require more than most. Some people are

153

like that. You can give it every half hour if needed."

I walked Marcia to the door. She was a damn good nurse. She'd stayed with us for over two hours. She'd arrived to find Dad in pain and distress, and she'd stayed as long as it took to make him comfortable. Unlike the encounters I'd had with the doctors and nurses at St. Mark's, there was no sense she was in a hurry. There was only the sense that she cared. She had told me that she found hospice nursing to be satisfying. I understood better now why she felt this way. She found the job satisfying because she genuinely cared.

Standing at the door, I gave her a hug. She hugged me back—a real hug, a firm, unhurried hug that said, *Trust me, I'm here for you. I won't let you down. And, most of all, I won't let your dad down.*

XVI. The Talk

Day 5.

I thought he would die during the night. At the 3:00 AM turning, he did not look well. His breathing was fast, and he was difficult to rouse. He barely opened his eyes as I turned him. He felt hot to the touch. Fever? I suspected the pneumonia was back. I held off on the morphine and the Ativan; he didn't need it—he was barely conscious.

At 5:00 AM, he looked even worse. His breathing was still fast, and his pulse felt thready and irregular. The small amount of caramel-colored urine in his catheter bag had not changed in volume over the last twelve hours. He was no longer making urine. His kidneys had shut down due to dehydration, and he was no longer eliminating the toxins building up in the blood. The advocates of terminal dehydration consider this to be a good thing. The toxins would act as natural anesthetics, and this would lead to a more peaceful death.

He barely responded during the turning, and again I held off on the morphine and Ativan. I sat in the chair next to his bed and watched him for about twenty minutes. I started to nod off. I wanted to stay with him, but I couldn't stay awake. I went back to bed, thinking he might well die while I slept.

At seven o'clock, my alarm sounded. I lay in bed and listened for the sound of his breathing. Nothing. I got out of bed and approached his bedroom with trepidation. What would I find? Would he be alive or dead? We'd brought Dad home to die, and out of compassion I'd hoped the dying would come sooner rather than later. Nevertheless, I felt a great sense of dread as I approached the room. I'd seen people die a number of times in my job as a physician, and I could deal with seeing death. But this was different. This was my father. My heart was racing. I was shaking.

Walking down the hall, I could see him lying there in bed, completely still.

Then, as I reached the bedroom door, I heard it: the soft, gentle sound of regular breathing. I entered the room, and looked at him in the morning light. There was a slow, regular rise and fall of his chest. Not only was he alive, he looked as peaceful and tranquil as a sleeping baby. I went to the bedside and took his hand and felt his pulse: strong and regular.

Tough old guy, I thought. Death had seemed to be closing in on him just a short while ago. Now death had retreated and was nowhere in the room. My father was thumbing his nose at death. He was sleeping and comfortable. I hated to wake him up and turn him, but the menace of bedsores outweighed my desire to leave him to his placid slumber. I gently shook him. His eyes opened, and I saw the sparkle of consciousness there.

"Good morning," I said. "Turning time. We'll make it quick, and I'll let you get back to sleep."

I went through the drill, pulling out the pillows, rolling him over, propping him, stuffing the pillows back under. He barely groaned, just a little grunt as I rolled him onto his side. He hadn't received any morphine in the last eight hours, yet he seemed to be in no pain whatsoever. Perhaps what they said about the sedating ketones and esters was true. Should I give him a small dose of morphine now, just to keep some in his system? I didn't want to enter the room in another two hours and see him writhing in pain. I decided to hold off, however. It was a chance, but it seemed like the right thing to do—leave well enough alone.

Arnold came at 9:00. As before, he bathed Dad, shaved him, and washed his hair. I had breakfast while Arnold worked his magic. As before, I took my cereal and coffee outside to the backyard patio. Before sitting down, I tossed a couple of handfuls of fish food to the koi in the pond. There were perhaps ten fish, and they came to the surface and gobbled the food voraciously. I watched them eating, refueling themselves, stoking the vital fires of life, then I went to the patio and sat down. It was a beautiful morning, cool and pleasant sitting under the cottonwood.

After breakfast, I went back into the bedroom. Arnold was just finishing up. Once again I was thoroughly impressed by how good Dad looked, freshly shaved and groomed. There was a difference, however, from when Arnold had first visited two days ago. My dad was visibly weaker now, no question about that. His cheeks were more gaunt and pale. His lips and skin were drier, more wrinkled. Arnold, bless his heart, was talking to Dad as he worked. Dad seemed to look at him as he talked. He knew Arnold was there. He was still conscious.

I walked Arnold out to the front door.

"The sore spot on his back is looking a little redder," Arnold said. "I put some more powder on and covered it with a dressing. I'll let Marcia know."

I let out a frustrated sigh. "I don't know what more I can do."

"There's nothing more you can do," Arnold said. "You're doing your best. It's so hard to keep pressure off that one area."

Arnold said he would be back in two days. I wondered—would he? Would Dad survive another forty-eight hours?

I went back into the bedroom. I was amazed and happy to see my mom was there, sitting in the chair next to the bed. She was holding Dad's hand in silence. She'd spent so little time with him since he'd come home. I walked over and gave her a hug. I pointed out, once again, what a good job Arnold had done. My mom agreed but then turned and looked at me with a look of concern.

"He's breathing so fast," she said.

I watched Dad breathe for a moment. She was right: his respiratory rate was up again, around forty. Just an hour ago, before Arnold arrived, the rate had been twelve. This was becoming a common theme: Dad's breathing rate seemed to vary wildly. Why so high now? Was he in pain? Arnold had said the bedsore looked redder. I scolded myself for not having given him a morphine dose earlier. I should have just kept the morphine going around the clock. I looked at Mom.

"I think he's due for his next dose of pain medicine," I said.

I got the medicine bottles, and my mom watched as I gave Dad the drops under his tongue. I sat down on the arm of her chair. After a moment, Mom looked up at me and said something unexpected, even bizarre. "He's had a stroke," she said.

My initial inclination was to say, *Hello, that's what this is all about, Mom!* Fortunately, I held my tongue. The enormity of what was happening—I knew she was not thinking clearly.

"Yes," I said. "He's had a stroke."

"And there's nothing they can do for it," she added.

"No," I said. "They can't. Nothing except make him as comfortable as possible. That's what we're doing. That's exactly what we're doing."

*　　*　　*

That afternoon I received an email from George Hansen, a good friend of mine. I've known him since our days together during medical residency. He and I had exchanged several emails since the stroke. I'd been keeping George updated on events, and he'd been sending me words of sympathy and support. George's latest message included the following piece of advice: "Before your dad dies, Chris, and preferably while he remains conscious, have that talk with him you've always wanted to have but have been forever putting off. You know what I mean. Tell him the things you've always wanted to say to him—the things you *need* to say. Now is your last chance to take care of that unfinished business. It's important. You won't regret it."

I thought about George's advice. I'd heard the stories of catharsis told by people who'd had the "talk" George was referring to. And I'd heard the stories of regret told by people who had *not* had the talk, people who had waited until it was too late. Dad and I had never been on "touch-feely" terms. Sadly, I could not recall ever having said, "I love you" to him, and I could not recall him ever saying those words to me. It just wasn't the way we interacted with each other. We expressed our feelings indirectly by actions rather than words.

At two o'clock, I turned him, suctioned him, wiped off his face, and moistened his lips. He was not looking so well again. His breathing rate was still up, and there were beads of sweat on his forehead. He felt hot. It had to be pneumonia, I thought. "The Old Man's Friend" had returned, as predicted by Dr. Wilber. He appeared weak. He was no longer moving his left arm in that agitated and disturbing way. He was quiet now, lying on his side, propped up on a pillow. Yet he was awake, and there was no question he was conscious. He tracked me with his eyes whenever I positioned myself in his field of view. His eyes would fix on mine and engage me whenever I spoke.

159

I lowered the bedrail, and, sitting in the blue chair, I leaned against the side of the bed. I took hold of my dad's left hand. I sat in silence for a minute, squeezing his hand and looking at his face and his eyes. I recalled what George had said in his email. "It's important. You won't regret it."

I started with the tricky stuff. Dad and I had not had a great many conflicts over the years, but there had been a few. Consequently, there were a few "I'm sorry-s" to get out of the way.

"There're some things I want to tell you, Dad," I started out. "Things I probably should have said a long time ago. But…you know how it goes. There are things you should say, but somehow you never do. So…. First of all, about those haircuts…." I laughed. He looked back at me. I do believe he was listening, and I do believe he understood.

"Seems so silly now, I know. But, boy, did we have some knockdown battles over my hair. So crazy. I wanted it long; you wanted it short. And, so, we fought and fought. That one time you dragged me to the barber and told him to give me a 'Marine cut'—remember that? Man, I was so angry, and I said I hated you. I must have been—what?—thirteen. I hated the way I looked with that Marine cut. I don't think I spoke to you for a month. My hair was so important to me back then. You know, teenage angst. Well, that was a long time ago, and my hair isn't quite so important to me now. But that was back in the '70s, back in the days of the counterculture and the hippies. Long hair represented all the things you were against: drugs, irresponsible behavior, a rejection of the world your generation had built. It was a path you didn't want me to go down. You were trying to look after my best interests. It all seems incredibly petty and unimportant now. But back then it was a big deal. So, I just want to say I'm sorry. Sorry for the battles.

160

Sorry for the things I said in the heat of my teenage narcissism and vanity."

He stared at me, his eyes fixed on mine. I wiped a few beads of perspiration from his forehead and repositioned the damp washcloth on it. I gave his lips a moistening. I continued.

"I'm also sorry about the fights we had over my marrying Sandy. She's Asian, and that was hard for you. It was the norm of your generation. White people married white people. Asians married Asians. That's just the way it was during your time. It's a prejudice, but it's a prejudice everyone had. If you'd been born twenty years later, it probably never would have been a problem. Fortunately, you came to accept Sandy over time. She's an incredibly good person, and I know you can see that now."

I squeezed his hand. He was listening.

"I'm also sorry about the grandkids. The grandkids you never had. Sorry because I know that's something you wanted very much. It doesn't look as though Lori will have kids either. Consequently, the Stookey clan will end with Lori and me. I know that's a disappointment to you. A big disappointment. It was a choice Lori and I had to make on our own, and—at least in my case—it was the right choice for Sandy and me. We love kids, but Lord knows there are enough people in the world—so, one or two less humans crowding the planet isn't going to make the world stop spinning. Still, I know how you feel, and I'm sorry for the letdown. I hope you'll forgive me on that one."

I stopped for another moment. That was it for the "I'm sorry-s." Now I turned to the 'thank you-s."

"I also wanted to say thank you—for a whole lot of things, a million things. Man, where do I begin? Thanks for

161

fathering me. I guess I'll start with that—a pretty important event in my life, you could say. Thanks for being a good dad. Thanks for working so hard to bring me up in a safe, well-provided household. Thanks for sheltering me from the hard knocks you knew so well when you were a kid growing up. You gave me everything I needed to grow up safe and strong. Thank you.

"Thanks, also, for teaching me the value of hard work. I know it's an ethic you learned out of necessity. I never faced that necessity, but you taught me the lesson all the same. It's a good lesson. There's nothing like honest, hard work to give one dignity and a sense of meaning in life. Thank you.

"Thanks for teaching me the value of truth. You were always one to question the premise of things and to look at the world through the eyes of reason. You have such a great love for science, and you passed that on to me. Science has greatly enriched my life, from the way I look at things every day to the way I work out my deepest philosophical beliefs. Science adds a hundred different levels of meaning to life, when I look up at the sky at night or when I just look at a tree in the backyard. What a great gift, Dad. Thank you.

"And thank you for the fun things we did together. So many things. Thanks for teaching me how to ride a bike, how to swim. For some reason, I always remember the time you took me swimming in the ocean at San Clemente—remember?—and the waves were so big. Scary big. You had me hang on to your neck as we swam out. I felt utterly safe as we went out through the waves. You told me to hold my breath and hang on as we dove under the waves. You were a damn good swimmer, and nothing could hurt us. Nothing. For some reason, I always remember that day. One of my best memories. Period.

162

"What else? Thanks for taking me hunting and fishing and hiking. I never became the hunter or the sportsman you probably wanted me to be, but I learned to love nature from you. That was such a great gift—another gift that enriches my life every day. Who needs a three-hundred-channel cable TV when you can watch the sun rise or hike along a mountain stream or just look up at the sky at night and ask, 'What's up there?' Nature—nothing touches it in beauty. You taught me that. Thank you.

"Thanks for putting me through college and med school. And thanks for turning me loose on my own after that. I remember once telling a friend: 'My dad gave me everything when I was young and paved the way for me until the day I became a doctor. Then he turned me loose. Since then, although he's a wealthy man, he hasn't given me a dime. And that,' I said, 'is exactly as it should be.'

"Thanks for being a faithful and good husband to Mom. So many people I know have childhoods torn apart by family problems and divorce these days. That darkness never fell over our house. You were always a good-looking man, and I'm sure you could have strayed—if you'd wanted to. But you opted for a good marriage over self-indulgence. You must be doing something right, Old Man, because she still loves you, you know, deeply, no diminution after sixty years, no cooling off since that love-at-first-sight moment all those years ago at the Navy dance.

"And, finally I guess, thanks for the more recent things, the little things and the big ones. Thanks for letting me visit your ranch whenever I wanted—what a great place and what a great gift. Thanks for the dinners you've made recently when I've stopped by. You've become a pretty good cook, you know. I have to admit, you make a damn good bowl of chili."

163

New beads of perspiration had formed on my dad's forehead. I wiped them away. I stood up and took the washcloth to the bathroom, rinsed it with cold water, and wrung it out. Folding the cloth in thirds, I brought it back into the bedroom, and placed it again on his forehead. I sat back down in the blue chair. I held his hand.

"There's one other thing, Dad. It's…it's something I've never said much. It's something I've never really said at all, actually. I've never said it because it's not our way. You get used to not saying it, and that's a bad thing. You should never get used to *not* saying something you *should* say, especially something you feel and believe."

I looked into those attentive eyes, those eyes that I knew were watching me. Absorbing me.

"I love you, Dad," I said.

I lifted his hand and pressed it against my cheek. For the first time since he had come home—for the first time since I'd walked into the ER at St Mark's and had seen him lying in the bed paralyzed and unable to speak—I began to choke up. My throat tightened, and my vision blurred as my eyes started to tear up.

"There. That wasn't so hard," I said, my voice quaking a little. "I love you. I love you." Saying those words, so daunting after so many years, suddenly seemed like the easiest thing in the world. Why had I waited so long? How is it we forge these steel barriers to expression? How and why? Thank you, George Hansen. I will be forever grateful for your advice. *"Have that talk. You won't regret it."* I stood up, kissed my father on the forehead, and I hugged him.

"I love you," I said again, savoring the words and the feeling the release from a fifty-year-old bad habit. "I love you. I love you."

XVII. Into That Good Night

Day 6.

Sometime during the night, he began to slip in and out of consciousness. At the three o'clock turning, his unblinking, half-open eyes had a glazed look. The eyes no longer tracked me the way they had before; they only stared blankly ahead. There was no moving of the arm, no moaning, no reaction of any kind when I rolled him over.

When I went in to turn him at 7:00 AM, he looked awful. He was breathing at fifty breaths per minute. His hands and feet were cold and had a bluish color. His pulse was fast and weak. He did make smacking movements with his lips when I moistened them. It was probably just a sucking reflex, however; it didn't necessarily mean consciousness.

Moreover, there was now a "rattle" sound associated with his breathing. Despite having seen death before, I hadn't fully understood the meaning of the term "death rattle." I knew it was a breathing noise people sometimes made just before they died—a gurgling sound from deep down in the throat where fluids collect when a person completely loses all swallowing and cough reflexes. Up until now, Dad's cough reflex (different from the gag reflex) had remained intact. He had coughed up his secretions as they collected in the back of his throat. However, the cough reflex was gone now. The secretions simply pooled in his throat, and the sound my father made as he breathed through those secretions was the death rattle.

I hated the noise. There was something chilling about it. It was the sound of a man drowning. I tried to make the sound go away by suctioning out his mouth secretions, but the fluid was too deep. I couldn't reach it with the suction catheter.

I knew death was near. I sat down in the blue chair and waited.

Late in the morning, Mom came into the room. She sat down in the blue chair and held Dad's hand. "What's that noise he's making?" she asked.

Of course, I didn't call the noise by its name. "It's from the secretions in his throat," I said. "I tried to suction them out, but I can't."

"I don't like it," she said.

"I don't either."

The rattle was too much for her. Without saying anything more, she left.

* * *

Lori came by in the afternoon. Like Mom, she asked me about the rattle. It was even louder now. It dominated the room. It was easy to see Dad was no longer conscious. The life had gone out of his dull, desiccated, half-open eyes. I left Lori alone in the room, so she could say goodbye in her own way. Like Mom, she stayed only a short time. She came out to the living room where I was sitting with Mom. Lori no longer voiced any reservations about what we were doing. It was plain to see that talking options was pointless now. Dad had passed the point of no return.

* * *

Marcia arrived at 4:00. She poured a can of Ensure for Mom, then she and I went into the bedroom. Despite the way Dad looked—unconscious, glazed eyes, the rattle—Marcia

166

went about her usual routine of comfort measures: moistening his lips, placing a freshly dampened washcloth on his forehead, suctioning, fluffing his pillows. She checked the bedsore. It was now a blister, one inch across surrounded by a red area. She gently washed the area, applied some powder, and covered it with a dressing.

All the while, she talked to Dad, despite his lack of responsiveness. "Hi, Bill." "Let's freshen up that washcloth." "I'm going to suction you out a bit." "Let's prop your head up a little—how's that?"

In addition, she gave him a dose of morphine. She reviewed my medication log and saw I hadn't given him any drugs in several hours. I hadn't seen the need. Screwing open the cap on the morphine bottle, she said, "I usually err on the side of keeping the morphine going," she whispered to me. "We don't know for sure what he feels right now."

As was her custom, Marcia gave my dad a hug before she left. "Goodbye, Bill." She did not, however, say "see you tomorrow," as was her custom. She knew. She knew she was saying goodbye for the last time. As a last kind act before leaving, she made sure the table fan was blowing properly over his face. Then we walked out of the room.

Out in the hallway, where Dad could not possibly hear us, she said: "We're getting close."

"I know."

"Are you okay?"

"Yes. It's what I want."

"I know." Marcia gave me a hug. "And you know what? It's what he wants, too."

I sat with him through the rest of the afternoon. Every two hours, I turned him and gave him morphine, even though I was nearly certain he was beyond feeling. I knew there was a good chance he would die sometime that evening or during the night, and I'd resolved to sit up with him all night if necessary. I wanted to be present when it happened. I did not want him to die alone.

The hard breathing continued. The rattle continued, louder. His hands and feet were now blue and cold to the touch, but his forehead remained fiery hot.

I sat in the blue chair, and I waited into the evening. I watched the hard work of his rapid breathing. Every ten minutes, I wiped away the beads of perspiration on his forehead. His body was working hard, fighting: the fever, the perspiration, the rapid heart rate, the struggle for air. And the rattle, the ceaseless rattle.

Dad was not dying the quiet, peaceful death I had hoped for. As I wiped the perspiration from his forehead, I found myself thinking of the famous lines from the Dylan Thomas poem:

> *Do not go gentle into that good night*
> *Old age should burn and rage at the close of day;*
> *Rage, rage against the dying of the light.*

Dad was, indeed, raging: burning with fever, breathing through the death rattle, hanging on to life. This is not what I wanted.

"Let go, Daddy," I whispered. "Stop the rage. Let go."

*   *   *

Sometime just before 10:00 PM, Mom entered the bedroom. Why she'd chosen that moment is unclear. She'd come in from the living room where she'd been alternately

168

sleeping on the sofa and watching TV. I stood up and offered her the blue chair, expecting she would refuse the seat—most likely she was just stopping by on her way to the bed. To my surprise, Mom stayed.

"Do you want to sit with him for awhile?" I asked.

"Yes," she said.

"Mind if I go to the kitchen and get something to eat?" I asked. I had missed dinner. "I'll be back in ten minutes. Will you stay with him?"

"All right," she said. "I'll stay."

I went to the kitchen and made a pot of coffee in preparation for the night vigil. I also made a quick sandwich and swallowed it down. When the coffee was ready, I poured myself a cup and sat down at the kitchen table to drink it. I had a long night ahead of me, and it was a relief to be away from the rattle for just a little while.

Just as I finished my coffee, Mom came into the kitchen. I figured she was coming in to say goodnight. I stood up, ready to head back into the bedroom. However, she had not come in to say goodnight. She had a concerned look on her face.

"Chris," she said, "your father—his breathing is so funny. Will you come?"

"You mean, fast?" I asked.

"Not fast," Mom said. "Funny."

I went quickly to the bedroom with Mom close behind. We went directly to either side of the bed. Dad's face looked very pale. His lips were an almost perfect blue. His dull, glazed eyes stared straight ahead and did not seem to heed our presence.

Then, at that very moment, just as we stepped to the bedside, he took his last breath. It was a small gasp—a sudden, brief inhalation followed by a little, half-exhalation. Then, he

169

was still. Perfectly still. The rattle was silenced. His vacant, frozen eyes stared into nothingness.

I grabbed his hand and waited to see if there would be another breath.

All of a sudden, without willing it, time stopped and my mind flashed back once again to the time my father and I went swimming in the ocean at San Clemente. I suppose it is my favorite memory of him, and in that instant I relived the memory one more time.

Twelve-years-old. A hot, sunny day. The air is full of the salty smell of the ocean. The waves are large and breaking hard. Dad, pulling off his shirt and tossing it in the sand, says, "Come on, let's go!" We both run out into the water and dive under the white-water of a broken wave rushing to shore. We begin swimming out, my father just ahead of me. As we reach the break zone, a large wave brakes directly on top of me, and it tumbles me under the water. When I come up to the surface, I am disoriented and a little frightened. But my father is right there next to me, and he sees I am afraid. "Put your arms around my neck!" he shouts. "We'll swim out beyond the break line, and then it's easy." I grab his neck, and riding on his back he swims out, his strong strokes pulling us rapidly out beyond the breaking waves. I feel utterly safe because I trust my father, trust him completely. When we get outside the breakline, I let go of his neck, and we tread water together safely beyond the breakers. We both laugh. Forming a water scoop with my hand, I splash my father in the face with seawater. He smiles and splashes me back, and we fall into a splashing war, the golden spray of ocean drops raining down over us under the brilliant sun.

There would be no next breath. It was as though he'd waited for us, waited for us to return before the final letting go. He knew how bad we would feel if we failed him and let him die alone. It was a final act of kindness to his family. His hand, blue like his lips, was ice cold. I didn't even bother to check for a pulse. I knew.

"He's gone," I said in a choked whisper, looking over at Mom.

"Gone?" she asked, sounding surprised. I don't think she'd understood how, through the day and the through evening, he'd been so close. She hadn't been expecting it the way I had. "How do you know?" she asked, her voice quivering.

"He waited for us," I said. "Just as we walked in. His breathing. He waited for us. Then he let go."

I walked around the bed and put my arms around her. There were tears in her eyes, but, to my surprise, she didn't break down and lose control. I hugged her as we both looked upon my dead father in silence. He did not look "at peace" the way death is sometimes described. I wish I could say otherwise, but he did not look at peace. His mouth, outlined by the ghastly blue lips, was half open, and a small amount of thick, white-green saliva hung from one corner. The NG tube that we had never used was still in his nose—it appeared somehow ridiculous, even grotesque, now.

And there was the look on his face. It was the same look I'd observed for the last few days—that look of perplexity, that look of bewilderment. The look was now frozen on his dead face. It was a look that I think will haunt me for the rest of my life. It will haunt me because I think I know the meaning.

Where, Son—my doctor Son—where was my hemlock?

171

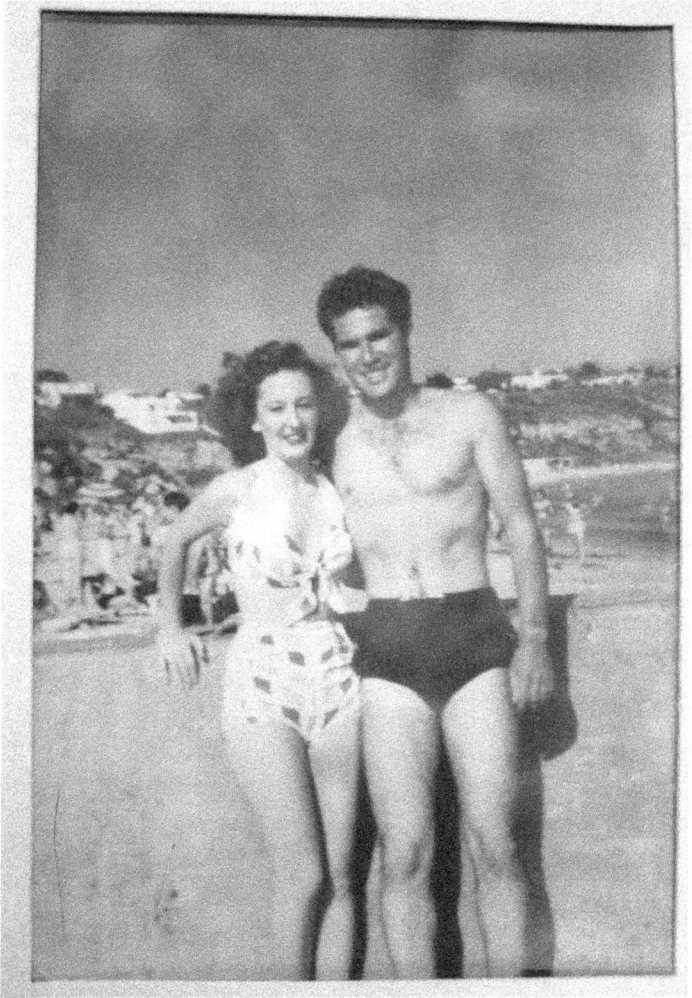

ALSO AVAILABLE BY CHRISTOPHER STOOKEY

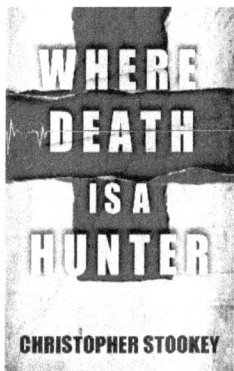

"[A] well-thought-out medical thriller [that] drew me in from the first page and had me hooked until the end. [A] cast of dynamic, believable characters and a plotline rife with tension and suspense…. Un-put-down-able."
—S.J. Pierce, author of *The Alex Rayer Chronicles*

"An intense medical thriller filled with corporate cover-ups, ethical dilemmas, and delightful twists and turns woven in for good measure. [D]eeply rich and realistic characters. [A]n absolute delight to read."
—Jennifer Higgins, Rundpinne Reviews

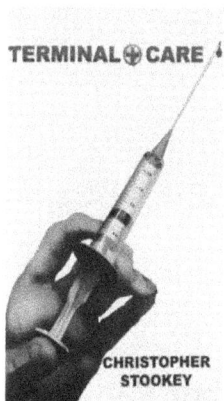

Available wherever books are sold or at www.SilverLeafBooks.com

www.ingramcontent.com/pod-product-compliance
Lightning Source LLC
Chambersburg PA
CBHW022038190326
41520CB00008B/636